MADISON CAMPUS

CANCER *What's It Doing In My Life?*

By Mary Alice Geier

* * * *

The Butterfly Connection

CANCER

What's It Doing In My Life?

A Personal Journal of the First Two Years of
Chemotherapy in the Career of a Cancer Patient

Mary Alice Geier

HOPE
Publishing House
P.O. Box 60008
Pasadena, CA 91106

Library of Congress Cataloging in Publication Data
Geier, Mary Alice, 1919–
    Cancer : what's it doing in my life?

    1. Geier, Mary Alice—Health. 2. Lymphomas—
Patients—Biography. 3. Cancer—Patients—Biography.
I. Title.
RC280.L9G454 1985   362.1'9699442 [B]   85–17559
ISBN 0–932727–05–0

Foreword

Mary Alice Geier's cancer career reminds me of a sign my husband's 74 year old secretary keeps over her desk that says: "Old age is not for sissies!" Neither is cancer for sissies.

All through our society are valiant people struggling with this stubborn disease. Many are patients, but there are others—doctors, scientists, nurses, therapists, volunteers—who struggle also. They share a common goal: the defeat of cancer.

Mary Alice leads us through days we each hope we will never have to live. She shares her inner struggle to be whole in spirit even while she lives with a body under attack. Her insights help us to understand what it is like to be a cancer patient, to view chemotherapy as the friend in battle rather than the enemy, to see the need we must share to befriend and support the friend or lover through the struggle.

As I write these words, Mary Alice Geier sits at a telephone responding to calls from cancer patients, their friends and relatives. She is a volunteer on the Cancer Information Service hotline, and she has come to the hotline today straight from the oncologist's (cancer physician) office not knowing what effect her chemotherapy will have today. She jokes and laughs. She empathises with the callers. And she struggles with her particular type of cancer.

Cancer is not for sissies. Mary Alice is not a sissy, but a strong, enthusiastic woman who daily chooses to live life as fully as possible. This is herstory at its best, told by an inner eye witness. Reading it will make you a better person.

—***Ruth Truman***, Ph.D., Director
Cancer Information Service of California

Acknowledgements

A constant companion during the journey this book records
has been my husband, Vance, also an ordained minister, now
retired. My illness brought him out of retirement to be
associate pastor, so that I need not retire from my parish duties
during the treatment period. His vocation during this period
became the care of his spouse, and no tribute can ever match
the extent of his love translated into practical nursing,
household management, chauffeuring, and consoling. Love is
indeed a many-splendored thing, calling forth skills and
stamina that made a co-ministry of the business of getting well
again.

This treasured partnership has extended to the practical
aspects in the preparation of this volume, for which I also
thank Vance. He is a "great pair of legs"!

Both of us have been overwhelmed and upheld by the
kindnesses of family and friends through the living of these
days, and by their encouragement for us to tell the story. To
name them all here would fill more pages than are before you.
We continue to bless our medical team, the nurses at Memorial
Hospital of Glendale and the counselors there who worked
with the We Can Do group.

We are humbled and inspired by the active praying on our
behalf in many circles of faithfulness.

—Mary Alice Geier

Table of Contents

Dedicated to the congregation of the
UNITED CHURCH OF EAGLE ROCK
who struggled along with their pastor
to rise up on wings like eagles,
to run and not get weary,
to walk and not faint!
and to the
participants in We Can Do
at Memorial Hospital of Glendale,
1983-1984
whose tears and fears
and hilarity and hopes
mingled with our own for
mutual support.

Introduction

Cancer: What's it doing in my life? No one in my immediate family has had cancer. I do not smoke, use alcohol, hormones like estrogen, have not been exposed to toxic chemicals in the work place. And like many people with only casual acquaintance with cancer patients, I never expected that it could happen to me. But here is the reality.

Behind me are almost three years of debilitating illness, finally diagnosed as "Progressive Lymphoma Stage 4", cancer of the lymphatic system. What is this doing to my life?

As a family we have weathered the changes in life-style abruptly thrust upon us when one parent became increasingly weak, partially disabled from the effects of chemotherapy. The familiar pattern of our lives has been reversed with a parent needing to take care rather than give it. In practical as well as psychospiritual terms, there has been deep drawing on the resources of faith, hope, humor and patience. Patience for a long haul.

In a conversation with a good friend, assessing the initial stages of this cancer career, I remarked, "At least I have learned patience." Her reply was, "Well, my friend, you have had to practice patience. It remains to be seen if you have learned it."

How well she knows me, the impetuous, eager-to-get-on-with-the-job me! But more importantly, how well she understands the dynamics of learning itself. In the field of human development, which is my teaching discipline, one can rarely find a textbook definition of "learning". More likely you will

1

read, "Learning has taken place when there is observable
change in structure, function or behaviour."

There you have it. Have I learned patience? Have I changed
in any basic way by becoming a long-term cancer patient? Are
there observable changes in my life's philosophy and purposes,
my priorities, my opportunities, my relationships, my interaction with my environment?

That's what this writing is about as I pursue the continuing
education career of being a cancer patient. I am an older
American, a partially-retired professional do-gooder. Is it too
late in life for me to learn patience?

I need to get these thoughts onto paper for my own learning
and growth. Yes, growth is still desirable—although we will try
by any means necessary and available to stop the growth of
those confused cancer cells that, through faulty genetic
information, don't have sense enough to stop growing when
enough is enough!

Growth is synonymous with change, just as true learning
means change. Cancer changes just about everything, and the
changes seem most undesirable. Yet some good things emerge
from the experience of a life-threatening illness. We will
celebrate many of those in this account.

I am grateful for the insight of one of our sons who burst out
with the affirmation soon after we were forced to accept the
dread diagnosis, "But, Mom, you're the same person!"

If I've learned patience, am I the same person as before? I
need to explore such questions, so the writing is part of my
therapy. It does not purport to be anything else.

You are welcome to come along on the journey. In all
probability, your life will be intimately touched by cancer
before long, in someone you love if not in personal experience.
The latest statistics indicate that one in three of us now living in
industrial societies stands in the path of this modern plague.

We need to know more about cancer just to cope in our
society. Cancer needs to come out of the closet as a subject for

conversation, if we are truly to understand and help each other. I eagerly read any account I find of the experience of other cancer patients. If our experience can provide encouragement for someone else's journey, there will be added meaning to the continuing struggle for me.

I've worked from journal notes and daily diary jottings to set down this organized journal of an impatient cancer patient trying to learn patience for what may be a long haul. The narrative portion covers the first two years of treatment. Some of the reflections in later chapters draw from experiences that came within six months beyond that, particularly material dealing with more professional involvements. Despite recurrence of the lymphoma after the first 18-month cycle of chemotherapy, and the discouragement of having to begin a new program of treatments, the future draws us along to new learnings and adventures.

"We" means myself and my spouse, Dr. Vance Geier, who has faithfully walked through this with me. I can speak, however, only for my own perceptions, to record as honestly as possible what cancer is doing in my life.

I am a minister by profession, but hasten to assure the reader that any resources of the spirit which have enriched my journey are available in equal measure to any sincere searcher. You should sense quickly my belief that learning is a joyous, religious experience!

Chapter 1

As Of This Writing

Life is organized just now around the chemotherapy treatment program. On the day I receive the injection, nothing else can be planned, for the drugs take over my body and my consciousness. I want to curl up in a ball, just get off the rolling globe until the aftereffects pass. Recently the appointments have been in the late afternoon, and I can pass through the slough of despond and suspended animation throughout the dark of night, rather than wasting precious daytime hours.

Currently the aftereffects are not severe compared to the earlier experiences. However, the memory of those former nights of wracking nausea are vivid, and I seem to hold myself ready for the worst to happen. So I emerge into the light of morning elated at my escape.

The minor symptoms that remind me that the drugs are at work include upsets in the gastrointestinal system, sores in the mouth, a bad metallic taste that lingers on, frequent cramping of muscles in legs and hands. I am aware that my kidneys are doing overtime to slough off the cancer cells destroyed by the drugs, even as my healthy cells reel, then repair and recover from the onslaught. Extra horizontal time is necessary, but my strength is not completely depleted in the two weeks before I return to the oncologist for a lighter dose (hair of the dog that bit me?).

Then there will be a month off! No needles, at least. I can hope for maybe three weeks out of every six to feel pretty good. Any special trips or entertaining, or dental work, can be scheduled during those three weeks. That's the predictable rhythm around which to build our family calendar.

I asked how many of these cycles are planned. The response was: ENOUGH.

The answer convinced me that we are in for a steady procession of these six-week courses. At least there is some stability to my career as a cancer patient for the time being, with pills of various hue maintaining systems control in between treatments. In contrast to the first series, my basic strength is building up rather than being drastically torn down by the toxic chemicals.

It seems strange, just at the time of adjusting to retirement, to have the rhythm for one's life programmed out predictably around health care realities. For so many years, it was our work schedules that determined the family calendar, and work responsibilities that set our priorities for the organization of time, talents and tenacity.

Even during the first two years of this illness, which curtailed much of my physical capabilities, it was my work that came first, insofar as strength allowed—and with the generous assistance of others who shared the load and spared me the walking. How much parish calling can be done by telephone when the caring community also adjusts to a grounded pastor! Preaching can be done from a sitting position on a kitchen stool when the legs are too weak for standing!

Now I have retired from the pastorate, although an active mind still thinks up sermon topics, and my loving concern surrounds former parishioners. I must learn a whole new rhythm for the living of these days. The restrictions of a chemotherapy treatment program provide a beginning structure. It has taken me these two years to accept that my body's special needs have *first* priority.

The surgeon who took my medical history before performing biopsy surgery recently asked, "Are you in good health?"

I reacted in disbelief, so he added, "Aside from the lymphoma, that is."

Aside from the chronic cancer, am I in good health? To have withstood the grueling treatment program for so many months, I must be basically of strong constitution.

I would like to be freed of chemical dependency. I wish I had full use of toes and fingers and leg muscles, that I could do aerobic exercises and play tennis and walk down into our orchard and back up again, that I could stoop over and get my hands dirty doing gardening. I would like to be cured of cancer. But in contrast to months of barely making it out of bed, I seem to be "in good health".

I can live with the present abilities and prospects. I can be more independent, while humbled by more continued dependency than I've ever had to accept.

Ironically, I'm now taking better care of this body, treating it with more respect than ever before in my life, even to religiously fastening the seat belt when riding in a car. Does it take a life-threatening illness to learn the importance of health care? Or to discover how closely related are health and happiness?

Are You In Good Health? I am in the best of health possible while harboring Progressive Lymphoma, Stage 4. Better to ask, *"Are You Happy?"*

I am eager for each new day, grateful for more leisure, the reduction of pressure from deadlines, the minimum of aches and pains. I am even grateful for the plan of treatment which outlines the possibilities for productive living and good fellowship with others within predictable expectations.

Indeed I am learning about healthy happiness and happy health. Was this trip necessary, this long training period for a cancer career? Healthy happiness is part of my reality. Maintaining that state is now my vocation. What preparation, what learning experiences, have brought me thus far on the way?

Chapter 2

Storm Warnings

We had returned from a mission study trip to Samoa, plunging into the hectic Easter season. Enthusiastically my husband and I were getting to the tennis courts early every other morning, taking walks to keep the muscles in tone, and attending an aerobics class twice a week. Those end of a semester deadlines always add stress, so there were reasons for feeling tired. The smog was at a level to bother anyone's breathing.

But something was different. Late in June there came a night of intestinal flu discomfort, with excruciating pain in the lower back. If there had been a fever, I would have phoned our doctor the next day. By the time I assessed this bout as something different, our physician was on vacation. I felt a tightening in the abdomen, yet no specific symptoms to propel me to see his standby.

Vance noted that I had lost my snore because my breathing was so labored during the night. A nagging suspicion began to accompany the increasing tiredness of my body and my breathing difficulty. Something must be seriously wrong in my system. Then I couldn't blow up the balloons for our daughter's birthday party. One Sunday I almost fainted before the sermon was finished, and had to sit down for a few minutes before closing the service.

8

A trip to the mountains would get us above the smog for a few days, and the drive was easy. But the higher altitude made it even harder to breathe, and with haste we returned to see our doctor's vacation substitute. His examination and the chest X ray noted an obstruction in the lung: either heart failure, an infection or a tumor—undetectable until the fluid could be removed.

The doctor agreed that we could visit friends that weekend as planned. I could not even walk a few steps in the sand near their beach house. By Monday the doctor noted, with some alarm, that I had lost six pounds in six days and that the X ray showed a large portion of the lung dark. He made no remark when I pointed out the swelling in the lymph nodes of my neck.

Our family physician returned the next Monday. As we got ready to go to his office, I packed a few things for an inevitable hospital visit. After all, they would have to drain off the liquid from the lung. Vance thought I was borrowing trouble by expectations of hospitalizations (that would confirm that I was really ill!), so we left the bag at home, then had to return for it and get to the hospital for my check in.

"Don't ever be an interesting case," our doctor had groaned when he examined me. Then, like an anchorman on a team, he began bringing in specialists to figure out the basic problem.

The next day, the chest expert drew off a liter and a half of fluid, and I could breathe again. I actually felt well as I went through test after test at the hospital. It was a week of rest. I was ambulatory and had lots of calls and visitors. With all that free time on my hands, I wrote a whimsical piece comparing the hospital to a resort hotel and gave it to the head nurse. It eventually found its way into the employees' newspaper and provoked some laughs (see Appendix I). Humor as therapy comes naturally to me.

But those tests turned out often not to be laughing matters. One paticularly horrid experience was having a needle inserted right into the fluid packet of the "pleural infusion" area to extract tissue for testing. Swords of fire sensations just above the diaphragm eroded any stoicism I could muster, and I gave out with some healthy screams. Victims of knife stabbings must lose consciousness almost immediately.

The chest specialist had stopped by my bed late the evening before to warn me. "I'm coming in the morning with a longer needle than before to snip some tissue," he said.

I sighed to myself, "Didn't they teach him any psychology in medical school?" Then I turned over and went to sleep, imagining myself on a rock in a mountain stream in Yosemite, reading all through a lazy August afternoon in the sun. Visualization also comes to my rescue naturally.

This specialist was also versed in tropical diseases. Could I have picked up some parasite during our South seas visit four or five months earlier? "Was there much kissing going on during that trip?" he wanted to know.

I avowed that I had been kissed by a Samoan chief! He was more interested in a scar I have carried since childhood when a bout with glandular fever caused my neck to be lanced. He theorized that what I had really suffered so long ago was tuberculosis and that my present predicament was a reemergence of TB, dormant since childhood. With my sister helping to jog my memory and confirm dates, I gave him information about the hospital in Iowa where there might be records of that illness, occurring in 1926. I signed releases allowing the specialist to write up my "interesting case" for medical journals.

Next a surgeon was called in to take a tissue sample from lymph nodes just below my neck. Our doctor explained that the diagnosis might well be lymphoma (he never used the term "cancer"). He told us about several of his patients who were dealing successfully with lymphoma through chemotherapy, projecting a hopeful attitude.

Intellectually I understood his words, but the idea of having cancer just did not register in my emotions. This was partly because the lab reports continued to find evidence of tuberculosis as well as evidence of lymphocytes—but never a clear-cut confirmation of one or the other.

We were just beginning to learn about how difficult diagnosis can be.

Whether or not the team of medics completely agreed, the convictions of the chest expert carried the day and he came to my bedside elatedly saying, "Congratulations! You have TB!"

Our reaction, too, was that of the three possibilities an infection seemed least threatening. An infection can be treated and cured. The medical team needed yet more test samples, however, and three days after the first biopsy, the surgeon was to reopen the almost-healed incision.

By this time I was suspicious that some of these procedures were more for their research than for getting me better. After more than two hours on the gurney waiting for the surgeon who was delayed by an emergency operation, I had worked myself into a Ralph Nader tizzy. Is this surgery really necessary?

Before going under anesthesia, I insisted on talking with the surgeon. When he sensed my agitation and near anger, he said, "We won't do it if you have any qualms."

Score one for patient autonomy and the right to participate in decisions, even though I had already signed the permission agreement paper. His explanation, however, of why they needed more evidence in order to prescribe treatment, calmed me.

I came out from under the anesthetic and the brief operation feeling euphoric, confident that now I could begin the road to recovery. So I was sent home to three months of invalidism, streptomycin injections every other day, and a collection of pills to be taken for a whole year. Though I was grounded, I was not infectious to anyone else. And I was curable.

True, I could not teach my fall class at the Community College, but I could give one-fourth time to my parish duties. Vance, who had recently retired from the ministry, was willing to pinch-hit for me for some of my parish duties. I offered to take a leave of absence, or to resign, but my doctor and my church counseled me just to go at a slower pace and to seek lots of help with my tasks.

How important this turned out to be for my morale. For one thing, it kept me from over-concentrating on my physical weakness. Weakness was the central experience—a bankruptcy of strength and energy. A few hours in the morning used it all up, and there was no reserve account on which to draw. I was overdrawn at the energy bank.

I wrote in the parish newsletter that month:

> *Exercise permitted to me includes lifting the telephone receiver, so we can keep in touch. Just remember, I'm supposed to be resting 75% of each day, so please ration your calls just as I shall have to ration and prioritize mine. The reality is that there is no reserve energy to tap into until medication and rest begin to make headway against virulent infection, focused in the lymph nodes. That may take a year ... Just remember, there may be fluid on the lung, but as of now there is no water on the brain. Please help me with the difficult discipline of resting when I would rather be up and doing.*

The nurse who came after his regular working hours to give me the shots every other day had been a student of mine in a church school class during his early teens. The renewal of friendship was good medicine. There was more than antibiotics entering my body with those injections.

I began the lessons in patience which were to stretch out into a lifelong learning course. A whole year before I could resume a normal pace of living. What a sentence! And yet how grateful I was for modern medicines. Just to breathe is not to be taken for granted.

Psalm 150 says it well: *Let everything that hath breath, praise the Lord.*

Chapter 3

Getting Better and Better?

Rereading what I had written in September 1982 reminds me of the undercurrent of anxiety during the first period of illness. Not knowing what is wrong is the most taxing part for patient, for physician, for family and supporters. Any symptom can be the signal for a number of dire diseases. At least we now knew the basic problem, or so we thought.

A year of semi-invalidism seemed interminable, yet we could work our lives around that. We have such faith in modern medicine that we seldom question our certainty that cure lies just around the corner—even if the block be extra long and progress be at a snail's pace. It now appeared to be a matter of directing our energies and marshaling our resources toward that goal.

Instinctively we knew the prayers of our friends to be a most precious and powerful resource. It seemed natural to let them know of our need for their support so we fell into the habit of issuing bulletins from time to time on the assumption that they cared. This assumption was reinforced by many expressions of love through letters and calls and proved to be the key to our own morale maintenance and the replenishing of our faith.

Such updates sent to scattered family and close friends were my journal efforts during that time of enforced idleness. Some excerpts from the one for October 4, 1982, indicate our perception of getting better and better:

The chest specialist says, "you're getting better." When he wanted to tap me again to remove a bit of fluid (I'm much like a sugar maple tree!), he could not pick up with his stethoscope where the pocket of fluid might be, and had to take me to the hospital ultrasound room to do the procedure. So, all the medication is making inroads into the pleural. By Thanksgiving time, I may be able to report being out of the woods, but probably as sappy as ever!

And by Thanksgiving Day, we had completed the streptomycin routine. I began experimenting with being up for more hours and doing more parish work.

As was our family custom on that holiday weekend, we composed the letter to be sent along with Christmas greetings to our wide circle of friends. It summarized what had happened throughout the year—communicating hope rather than anxiety. We mailed it the first week of December. By Christmas Day, we had a vastly different story to tell.

Chapter 4

Earthquake

Had the antibiotics aimed at conquering TB kept the underlying lymphoma in check? There is no medical reason for thinking that. Nevertheless, it was within three weeks after cessation of those injections that lymph nodes in my neck became swollen and sore.

Our doctor sent me to a surgeon for removal of one of them for testing. The biopsy was scheduled for the next week. By that time a large area in the left groin was enlarged and painful and feverish to the touch. It was like trying to hatch a dinosaur egg!

At the hospital, our doctor told me, "I'm sorry you have pain, but at least this tells us you do not have Hodgkin's disease where the nodes become swollen and the patient does not feel anything."

I had privately wondered if Hodgkin's disease could be my problem. Since I had always heard this was incurable, his words had the effect of relieving anxiety. (Actually, great strides have been made in the last decade in the treatment and cure of Hodgkin's disease.)

The biopsy was done on Thursday. The leading lymphoma expert in the country who is at USC Medical Center looked at the lab reports and still found this an "unusual case". By now they were definite about one thing: "We have a malignancy here."

15

So a bone marrow sample was needed and I made the acquaintance of the doctor who was to program my life for a long time to come—the oncologist on the team. He performed the unpleasant but bearable removal of bone marrow sample while I lay on my stomach on the hospital bed. Since it was Friday, the lab results would not be known until Monday.

We now knew there was a malignancy. Why did we not have an immediate reaction or even say the word "cancer" to each other? It had never occurred to me that I would ever have cancer. No one in my immediate family had ever had cancer. Bronchial problems had plagued me since childhood, and I sometimes remarked about all those childhood illnesses coming back to haunt me.

The tuberculosis diagnosis, unusual as it is in the 1980s, could be intellectually explained. But I had never visualized that I would be a cancer patient. Even on that fateful Friday, because there had been so much uncertainty for four months about the diagnosis of my present condition, I was still not compelled to "think cancer" until all the reports would be in, after the weekend. Cancer was just not going to cross my mind.

Meanwhile there was the weekend. Must I waste it in the hospital? A letter written on Christmas Day to family members summarized both the happenings and our mood:

> A biopsy of lymph nodes on the neck revealed "we have a malignancy here," hinted at in the August diagnoses. Apparently the TB was real, is now under control, and has masked the lymphoma. If we knew why, we'd have the Nobel Peace Prize.
>
> Next day a bone marrow test to see how extensive it is, what will be the proper dose of chemotherapy. But no lab work gets done on the weekend, so I asked for time off for good behavior, and our family doctor arranged for me to have a twelve-hour pass out of the hospital on Sunday, to preach, partake of potluck lunch, attend the Church Council meeting and the Christmas party for our

*neighborhood Board and Care Home residents ... What
a day! I checked back into the hospital, still in my long
skirt and holiday colors at 8:30 P.M.*

It had felt good to be doing my regular work and sharing in
pre-Christmas celebrations. There had been no time to think
about the implications of impending chemotherapy. While I
knew practically nothing about cancer, I had learned from
friends how disagreeable and devastating chemotherapy can
be. The term "lymphoma" had not been part of my vocabulary
before August and not one of the doctors ever used the term
"cancer".

Of course, we knew. We must have known the worst. But we
were in suspended animation until the lab results would be
reported—not deliberately suppressing the facing of what
cancer meant, just not entertaining any thought about it. For
the reality of cancer, there was as yet "no room in the inn" of
our mental residence.

It was not so much deliberately letting other thoughts of
Christmas joy and love and gratitude crowd out having to
think about cancer. It was more like the knowledge that a big
ship was riding at anchor out at sea which did not yet have
clearance to put into the harbor. We were harboring no
conscious thoughts about cancer at the moment.

Vance reports having looked up the meaning of lymphoma
when it was first voiced in August, then just hoping against
hope.

On Monday, Vance came early and stayed late by the
hospital bed, waiting to hear the doctors' report. The long day
passed with no visit from any one of the medical team. It
turned out to be a day for just taking up space, being in
limbo—a day for practicing patience if there ever was one. I
completed a book review I had been asked to write for a clergy
journal.

What was going on behind the scenes as the doctors
conferred? Is it so bad that they do not know what to do? The
silence was not comforting, indeed it was exhausting. It took

effort to keep anxiety from building up. We would rather know.

Tuesday morning, our physician and the oncologist appeared together with plenty of news to digest all at once. The diagnosis was "Progressive Lymphoma, Stage 4".

"What is the next stage?" I wanted to know.

"There isn't any."

That was the moment of truth, the shocker. When I asked, "What if I opt not to have chemotherapy?" there was an even sharper shock.

"There would be two or three months before the tissues would build up to destroy the function of the other organs."

Not even a split second was needed to opt for chemotherapy, despite all I had heard about that.

How positive the medics were about what chemotherapy could do for me. After all, Golda Meir had lymphoma for 14 years while carrying on as head of a modern state. A worthy role model, to be sure.

"We'll have you out on the tennis courts again," promised the oncologist—the only promise I have ever heard him make.

Through all of this traumatic half hour, my husband was making notes of the information and treatment plan being outlined. How glad I am for that practical gesture, for my reactions were less than pragmatic just then.

Then a feeling of complete exhaustion and dread took over. As Vance held me, I gave in to tears—grieving that our familiar way of life was over, if not forever, certainly for a long stretch of involve-ment with medical procedures. An earthquake was shaking our foundations!

I grieved that Vance would have to spend his retirement being burdened with my health care. I grieved that my capacity for doing the work of ministry and teaching might be abruptly taken away. Looking back, I cannot remember any flashing thoughts about mortality. The threat to continued life was not an overriding presence in those critical moments.

The doctors were so genuinely positive about their ability to control this kind of disease (without ever promising cure—oh, how careful they are not to project false hope). But life as we had been living it was definitely going to be drastically changed.

Thanks to Vance's foresight in taking notes, my spouse had something tangible to do as he left for home to type up the bulletin for our extended family, phone the children, mail out the letters, and rush back to be with me.

His memorandum follows:

Dear Friends—

Following is a summary of the present situation:
DIAGNOSIS: Progressive lymphoma, Stage 4, diagnosed from lymph node tissue and bone marrow sample.
TREATMENT: Chemotherapy: injections, one large and one small, eight days apart, every month, plus pills, for about 18 months. Dose may be reduced after about six months.
OUTLOOK: Favorable. The disease is treatable, as an outpatient after the first treatment in the hospital . . . Probably can carry on normal activity, depending on tolerance of treatment. The treatment she has been getting for the last four months for tuberculosis will continue, although that disease is pretty much under control.
POSSIBLE SIDE EFFECTS: Three main areas affected—
1) Hair probably will fall out, but will grow back again. (A woman in our church has gone through this, and her hair grew back; she is 87.)
2) Lining of the intestines; this is naturally renewed every three days, so no problem.
3) Bone marrow: The crucial area, since it produces blood cells and platelets. This will be carefully monitored.
4) Probably some nausea, but antidotes are available.
NATURE OF DISEASE: Can attack person of any age. One can be born with it. Cause unknown. Older people have better chance of recovery because general growth

*has slowed down. Patients treated for it have been
known to live a long life ... This kind of systemic cancer
is much easier to treat than the other kinds, and the
results are more "gratifying." It is not inherited nor is it
communicable.*

*Mary Alice is holding up quite well, though we both
had our moments of depression today. We know you will
keep us in your thoughts and prayers ...*

A major learning on this earthquake day was the basic need
to be in touch with loved ones, the utter dependence on the
network of relationships through which the Divine Love is
made manifest. To involve our support system was like
sending out a call for blood bank donations, knowing that
their prayers could generate power for our own persistence of
faith in being upheld by the Everlasting Arms.

Their caring undergirded our will to cooperate with the
medical treatments. Letting the network know was a positive
action toward cooperating in our own healing.

Chapter 5

Living With Chemotherapy - I

No doubt about it now, I had become a cancer patient. By late afternoon of Double D-Day (Drastic Diagnosis Day), the contents of seven vials were drip-dripping my first chemotherapy treatment into my veins from the overhead dispenser. The patient in the bed next to mine had a visitor who talked noisily and stayed too long for me to completely relax or give in to my own thoughts.

Our doctor came by, later than his usual rounds, sat down on the bed, sighed, and said, "How tired I am! It is very tiring to bring bad news to people."

His very human response endeared him to me even more, this good as well as competent physician—a proven source of strength and confidence over many years of our family's life.

The anti-nausea medication which the nurse added to the intravenous mix every so often through the night kept me from too much discomfort, but caused diarrhea which kept me in the hospital an extra day. I went home to pre-Christmas activity, buoyed up by prednisone pills and lots of tender loving care from family and friends.

The twelve days of Christmas flew by with many more than "five golden rings" of the doorbell and telephone. There were meaningful traditional services at the church, where I was able to take care of my responsibilities as pastor, interspersed with many hours of horizontal rest time.

A week from the first chemoptherapy dose I reported for the follow-up injection and was moved to write the following:

THE LAUNCHING OF AN OUTPATIENT

The first chemotherapy treatment was given in the hospital, at the end of a day when pathologists had come to agreement about a diagnosis which had been pending for months. The highs and lows of that day drained out most feeling or creative thinking. It was a night just to be endured.

Now, a week later, it was time for treatment number two. Already the swelling of the lymph nodes had subsided. I felt better and had almost mastered the regimen of tests, pills, potions and diet to regulate the biochemistry set my body had become.

There was natural apprehensiveness about the unknown. What would this treatment be like? How would I feel afterwards? Four days before Christmas, would I be incapacitated by this next dosage? Old wives' tales about the dire effects of these chemicals on one's system competed with the clinical optimism of my new doctor.

As a pastor, I had spent many hours next to the beds of those "dying of cancer", from an eleven-year old to an 80-year old First World War veteran; from contemporaries who were best friends to casual colleagues. But no one in my immediate family had given me a role model for this. Mine was the first such case.

What ambivalence I felt as I walked into the crowded waiting room of the oncologist to find myself a part of a democracy of people from all ages and conditions of life, persons in various phases of chemotherapy. There was a football-build teenager, pale and with thinning hair, whose mother's hand brushed his from time to time. Two women, scarves draped turban-style on their heads, animatedly compared notes in Spanish.

An elderly man emerged from the treatment room, teetering on crutches, carefully lowering himself into the too-low chair, obviously experiencing light-headedness. It was a melting pot in more ways than one, this room! And what a camaraderie could be felt.

A cheerful staff person would open the door to call someone's name to come in for some lab work; that person would return to wait some more. There was warmth and friendship radiating between staff and patients, and among the old-timers to the routine.

So this was to be a new community for me for the next year and a half! A community of those living with chemotherapy.

I was glad that I had dressed up for the occasion, even to wearing my holiday corsage. The cell growth that would be stopped by the chemicals would allow for growth in empathy and spiritual resources. When my name was called, I found that I no longer dreaded what was to come, but welcomed the miracle of the wonder drugs. I stepped inside not to begin a sentence but to claim my Christmas present, the gift of the promise of new life!

—Rev. Mary Alice Geier,
Los Angeles, December, 1982

THE BEGINNINGS OF A JOURNAL

This piece was the beginning of my journalizing. Every day since then I recorded in diary form the happenings, the callers, the special things to be remembered. Under seperate cover are the occasional reflections which trace more the inner journey. Up to now, the account you are reading has been primarily background material. Now I begin to put down the more important saga of learning to live with chemotherapy.

Yes, *live with* in the several meanings of that word: to continue to live with the help of chemotherapy, certainly. Very soon it became a matter of enduring, putting up with, living despite the effects of the treatment. At this point of beginning, I was putting up a brave front, thinking positively about the regimen laid out for me for the next year and a half.

Here is the beginning entry in my new journal:

> *This journal will be an entertainment center: the entertainment of thoughts, ideas, feelings, questions— some uninvited or even unwelcome. This Open House for thoughts could become as crowded as the living room where we attended a holiday party. No thoughts will be turned away, but not all will be encouraged to stay long. Some will be put up with rather than put up.*
>
> *For instance, once or twice there has drifted across my consciousness the What Ifs. What If this is my last Christmas? This question will not be given lodging at this time. No room in the inn for it just now.*
>
> *I shared with my family this question: Should I make an effort to get all my personal effects and affairs in order, albums and old letters organized, so that they would know where such things are, which have special meaning for me? Then I answered my question in the negative. It is not appropriate for now. There's too much involvement in the living present. Since I'm feeling better and more energetic than I've felt in months, my energies will be focused on today and a few immediate tomorrows.*

I was able to report in the January church newsletter:

> *The immediate effects of the first two treatments are positive: 90% reduction in the swelling of the lymph nodes in my neck and groin. I have a bit more energy for more hours of the day, although continuously aware of the weird and wonderful things going on in the bio- chemistry set that is my body ... we gratefully rest back on the net ropes of our support system of friends and relations. As we pray that the cancerous cell growth can be stopped in its tracks, we know that spiritual growth is increasing exponentially as we live out this adventure.*

The last journal entry of the old year reports:

> I heard my husband say in a telephone conversation,
> "We're not getting any younger." What an optimistic
> statement that now seems to me. Much better than
> having to say, "I'm not getting any older."

I had concluded that at this point I was not dying of cancer,
the unspoken fear, but living with chemotherapy, coping with
cancer. After all, those doctors had a stake in keeping me alive
through the treatment months to justify their confidence in
pharmaceutics!

And then came the second treatment cycle, and the internal
earthquake it caused. From my journal, these notes, written a
day or two after the injection:

> In the car coming home I could already feel the effects
> of the drug, much like in the hospital, not being able to
> fully concentrate or focus my thoughts. This continued
> through the afternoon . . . and the night was spent
> vomiting every hour on the hour, losing everything in my
> stomach, including all of the anti-nausea pills I had
> taken.
>
> It's a good thing I'm not an astronaut. The headline in
> today's paper reads "LOSING ONE'S LUNCH IN SPACE
> ISN'T MACHO". I am a bit spaced out, but no need to be
> macho about it. I've always had trouble with the first
> verse of "Amazing Grace," because I didn't consider
> myself a wretch, but it will be easier to sing it now. I was
> certainly "a-retch" for one whole night.
>
> I'll know how to handle this next time, because I do crawl
> out of the doldrums and start functioning again, 24 hours
> later. Even so, that's a lot of empty time for one who's
> supposed to be leading a normal life.

The oncologist emphasized leading a normal life, and I
wanted very much to comply. That included looking for the
humorous in any situation. Another entry caught the same
hopeful attitude about the chemotherapy treatments:

My appetite is returning. Losing one's lunch (plus) may not be macho, but 24 hours of it did knock off the pounds added due to holiday extravaganza and cheating on munchies. It will be easier to face the start of the next therapy cycle knowing that "this too shall pass," and I can look forward to feeling better within a couple of days.

My cheery optimism was encouraged by the evidence that the first treatment had worked so well on me against the tissue buildup, and also by the effects of prednisone which I took in pill form during the week between treatments. The effect of this hormone can be a heightened sense of well-being, restlessness and increase in energy. I was peppy, not so much a wet noodle as I'd been for months, more like Rice Krispies! I was on a high, very confident that I could handle whatever chemotherapy had to dish out.

January 6th journal entry:

If my hair is being zapped so fast by the chemicals, think what they're doing to those cancer cells to frustrate their division and growth.

Within the first month my hair had been completely uprooted. Becoming bald does something to one's self-image, but it was an anticipated reaction. Worse things could (and did) happen.

I had bought a dark brown wig, the color my hair used to be, while there was still enough of my front hair anchored so that I could brush it up over the hairpiece around the face, making it look quite natural. My daughter did not immediately notice that I was wearing a wig, and my daughter is one who notices everything about my appearance. I told a friend I'd found a way to get rid of gray hair, and quipped something about "died hair".

After several nights when the pillow became covered with hair, I began saving it in a plastic bag, so that I might match it for a custom-made wig. And then I was so bald that I could comb my hair (singular) with a towel.

One night as I was undressing, Vance walked in and was startled to see this creature, bald from the waist up, and for a moment thought some stranger was in the room, some creature from outer space!

Living a normal life meant that on the day after the milder treatment I conducted a funeral for a woman who had died of cancer. The work of ministry went on. There would be three weeks before the next needles. I thought I had learned to live with chemotherapy! My mind could now shift to reflections about having contracted cancer.

Chapter 6

Why Did Cancer Hit Us?

I had put off dealing with the possibility of dying from cancer, but related questions crowded the agenda of dealing psychologically and spiritually in the early days of being a cancer patient.

The question of *Why*, that overarches all reactions to a cancer diagnosis is followed hard upon by the question, *Why Me?* Although it is a completely normal response, I found that I did not entertain it for long, for I could just as well ask, *Why Not Me?* If a fourth or more of my contemporaries are facing cancer in this decade, why would I not also be a candidate? Even though the obvious known causes were not a part of my life-style, why should I be exempt from something hitting a wide cross section of neighbors and friends?

My husband had gone through the *Why? What Caused This?* stage already—four or five months before when I had taken ill so suddenly. At that time I was impatient with such questions, bending all energy just to meeting the crisis, doing what could be done to make a turnaround.

This reflects the varied ways different persons react in accepting illness in themselves or in others. Deep in our childhood training in traditionally religious families is that sneaking suspicion that if you get sick, it is your own fault. Or perhaps it is punishment of some sort.

Dr. Robert Bermudes in his book *Conquering Cancer*[1] has a chapter on sin and sickness which discusses this tendency. He notes for instance that good people are supposed to instinctively know the correct thing to do and be in control of themselves at all times. Thus illness must mean that one has not achieved self-mastery over one's own body or health care. Both a patient and the family members have to deal with some guilt feelings when a loved one gets sick. What did we do wrong? What did we fail to do?

Particularly as we understand more about the role of the immune system in preventing precancerous tendencies from being triggered, do we take more seriously the life-style factors, recognizing that failure to keep healthy, to avoid habits and stress situations which could lower resistance, all play a part?

Writers like Norman Cousins encourage us to be participants in our own treatment and healing, cooperating with medical treatments while adding psycho-spiritual components generated out of belief in our own responsibility. If we can have some such role in the healing process, it is logical to believe that we also participated in causing the illness.

A friend sent me *Getting Well Again*[2] by Drs. O. Carl and Stephanie Simonton—currently the best known documentation of how cancer patients can add their own healing powers "to normal medical treatments and increase chances of long-term, high-quality survival." I read it seriously, reflecting in my journal as follows (dated, February 2, 1983):

> *In the first section on what causes cancer cells to get started, most of the case studies don't seem to apply to me at all, except for the stress factors in the six to 18 month period before the onset, or the diagnosis.*

I then began to analyze various stress points, many related to my work, some specific troublesome incidents, the feelings of helplessness I had about the church. There had been family stresses, too, but I noted that

> *we did cope, refused to be victimized, and took the initiative to change the dynamics. Apparently it's the*

*way one copes that is more crucial than the stressful
situation itself... Could the failure of my immune system
to successfully turn back cancer cell growth date from
my acute diabetes onset in 1979? If so, my body did
make good adjustment, and diet change has been
effective. The move to a new house and a new work
position had come at the same time, yet it had been a
deliberately chosen move. In recent months, I've been
conscious of being too tired too often, yet physical
fitness has been a strong preoccupation all through the
year preceding this illness.*

The Simonton book suggests that emotional response to
stress can create susceptibility to disease, insofar as such
emotional stress can suppress the immune system, thus
shackling the body's natural defenses against cancer and other
diseases. The significant factor is how the individual copes
with stress.

"When coping techniques are faulty, one learns a lesson in
human finitude. We have only so much energy, no more. If our
life-style takes too much effort for dealing with the environment, we have less to spare for preventing disease." They quote
from a book published in 1893: "Idiots and lunatics are
remarkably exempt from cancer in every shape." It is those
who assume responsiblity for the feelings of other people and
take on the burden of helping people feel better, who are sure
to have stress.

Now we are getting on my case! And my reflections included
these thoughts:

*How can anyone who truly cares about other people
and the world keep from being stressed? All pastors
have a built-in susceptibility, because we extend this
sense of responsibility to the whole world! And how
about the extra stresses of being a woman minister?
When you're number two, you try harder! Yet I cannot
see myself caring less!*

Of course, the process of dealing or not dealing with stress successfully does not cause cancer, but permits cancer to develop. Simonton again: "Creating meaning of the events in our lives, we choose, not always consciously, how we are going to react. The intensity of the stress is determined by the meaning we assign to it and the rules we establish about how we will cope with stress." I could think of so many situations where no rules seemed workable, where I was damned if I did, damned if I didn't.

Continuing to delve into the Simontons' book, I tried to see where I fit in the discussion of personality type factors. They and others suggest that certain personality profiles may be more prone for cancer. I wrote at that time:

> I can't see these applying to me at all. But I shall be open to further understanding . . . I've run through this book quickly, and will return to it for careful use of the exercises on relaxation and visualization. But I want to test out first whether my instinctive coping attitudes are consistent with their planned progression of self-help and self-regulation.

Clearly I was stimulated by the material in this book, the first serious reading I had done on a holistic approach to cancer, and I tried discussing it with my oncologist on the next visit. What a strong reaction he had. "Pure quackery," he called it! "You can't think yourself well," and "no one knows what causes cancer. There are a hundred different kinds of cancer and a hundred different causes."

He also told me he was very distrustful of "Positive Thinking" because it can give you such a guilt trip. If you don't improve or get well, you blame yourself. I would guess his is a typical physician's perspective, because the various claims of quick cure schemes can lure patients away from the steady course of treatments needed for real control of the disease.

Some of the advertising of the Simonton book may give the impression that one can think oneself well, but the work in total emphasizes using positive attitudes and visualization exercises to augment, not to replace, medical treatments.

The problem of *What caused the cancer in the first place?* does not get settled easily. Does anyone know what causes an earthquake? Imperceptible changes and shifts deep within the earth, unfathomable and unmeasurable for the most part, go on for centuries and longer. There are some known fault lines from past geological incidents which increase vulnerability, but none of the sophisticated technology can yet predict when an earthquake will happen.

In the case of lung cancer, there is no doubt that smoking is a cause, yet not all smokers get cancer. Certainly a convergence of factors, differing with each individual, triggers the earthquake of a cancerous condition, very difficult to detect in early stages.

Everyone experiencing such an earthquake has a need to find the cause, to fix the blame for something which has happened to change the normal life-style. Be it pain, disease, disability, the death of a loved one or the loss of a job, the dynamics of the grief process over the many disasters we experience in a lifetime are similar.

Cancer plunges one into some grieving, because nothing will be the same again. Anger is an expected response, but did not rise to the surface for me, perhaps because I had worked out coping responses to anger-producing experiences already faced—including a sense of righteous indignation over much that happens in society! Reading the morning newspaper is enough to make me angry, but I can't afford to use up all that emotional energy, so I must be selective in my indignation.

I was on the edge of being angry at my medical team for taking so long to make a clear diagnosis. After all, should I not have started on chemotherapy three or four months earlier? The oncologist responded to this idea with assurance that the splendid way my system was responding now to the treatment meant no real time had been lost. And so trustful have I always been of the authority of modern medicine, I could not direct anger against my doctors.

Why cancer here? Now? Why me? These questions were far from solved. But there were other things to reflect upon along the way, and many more disagreeable treatments to endure.

Chapter 7

Who Am I Now?

With enforced rest came time for the mind to roam widely, time for much inner dialogue and prayer, which for me are closely related. Part of my resentment about the disorientation and instability I experienced some 24 hours after the intravenous injections was that I was robbed of those hours for deep thinking. I had a sense of urgency about getting thoughts organized.

Whatever might have been my fault in bringing on this terrible health crisis, I knew that my current vocaton was to sort out priorities and nurture attitudes that would help my body cooperate with the treatments. My spiritual life must operate at full speed. Along with my oncologist, I had a mistrust of "positive thinking" as a cure-all. I considered myself to be a reality-tester. So I could entertain almost any scenario of what might happen, but my commitment was to deal with each day's vicissitudes as they came.

As I looked into the mirror of what my life pattern had become—a cancer patient, weakened and disabled by chemotherapy—the problem of *Identity* presented itself. I confided to my journal "how important to my sense of identity it is that I can continue my work, thanks to Vance's help and the church's willingness for me to go at my own speed."

Speed was not the best image here! Actually, no one had ever been pushing me to be so busy. It was my own ideal of efficiency that kept me overreaching energies. But can one care too much? Can one live out the love ideal without overextending one's self?

There were points of conflict in sorting out a new sense of identity—that of a long-term patient:

This question of identity! How important all the family and old friends are in affirming my sense of who I am to them, regardless of present work. To be so affirmed as a lover/wife, mother, sister, pastor, friend is a daily blessing. Why should I be surprised? Vance asks. "That's what family means."

This illness has just released the expression of their love in such an energetic way, channeling so much strength to us. I bask in the love made manifest. No matter what, the MAG they know and love is intact—not totally invalid—and valuable and worth saving, regardless of my performance professionally.

Friendships from 40 years ago and more are fresher than springtime. My thought waves are literally alive and my memories clear as crystal. What a gift of healing and hopefulness each call and card brings. I'm the richest person alive.

As I come out upon the other side of these 18 months of chemotherapy, I should be able to retire more gracefully, because my identity will not be soley resting on MAG the minister and teacher, but just MAG the person, whose life interacts with so many others in so many spectra. I want to reach out and hug everyone, I want to delve more deeply and cultivate those friendly relationships. That's why I don't just now feel a need for a therapy group of new relationships.

My sense of identity is strongly linked with my vocational life, of course, so the messages of concern and prayer from colleagues of long and short standing are wonderful

*surprises. What a lot of constellations of comrades I
have. It will take a lifetime to let them know our
appreciation. The dear folk of our parishes, too . . .
knowing what they have lived through, to have them
hold us so dear is very humbling.*

*I sense that I have participated in my own healing by
reaching out to let the support system know what is
happening here. I made an assumption that they care,
and I certainly need their caring. Even so, the degree
and perceptiveness of their responses come as a
surprise, like rain from heaven. I'm just floating on a
cloud of supportive systems. I'm on the receiving end
and with little opportunity to reciprocate. This means
behavior modification for me—to be a passive recipient,
gracefully and gratefully, without feeling guilty that I
can't be the giver. That is a new wrinkle. It is blessed to
receive! Getting well will be my return of thankfulness.*

It is important to put these expressions of inner realities
alongside the near depression of other chapters yet to come.
Just as my blood count was on a yo-yo because of drug action
in my system, so moods also had ups and downs—but the basic
attitude was upbeat. What my Chinese pen pal calls my
"correct attitude", drawn from deep resources, was on the side
of healing.

Put another way, when I wrote about the four levels of
CT—as I had dubbed my chemotherapy:

First, of course, is the Chemical Therapy. *The chemicals
of the treatment are crucial to stop the growth of the
cancer cells. The whole regimen of diet and medications—to strengthen the immune system so it can
patrol, destroy and prevent the cancer from continuing—
is basic. I need to deal with the imagery of battle which
comes to the fore when you think of dealing with cancer.*

*Is this in conflict with my commitment to nonviolent
resistance to evil? Of course, I have been a fighter for
what I think is right—willing to fight when the outcome
was by no means likely to be favorable. How about*

fighting off cancer? The body's immune system is usually seen in that imagery—a lot for me to think about.

The second CT is Care Therapy, *administered primarily by Vance. How often he anticipates my needs, does the myriad errands, looks after me. I'm glad I can do most personal things for myself, but there's no way I could have managed without him and his unconditional love. What a partnership!*

Third, I could cite the Caring and Concern Therapy *of the whole family, plus the friendship web. If anything beneficial can be attributed to the experience of the last half year, it is the activation of this caring concern community—the richest asset for health and purpose in life.*

Fourth is Career Therapy—*having work which I can still do in large part, like Preaching, which gives such focus for my reading and reflecting, for personal prayer and theologizing. Having an outlet for sharing this process is a special blessing. I'm so grateful I was not forced to give it up.*

Teaching is in the same category. It is something I know how to do, so the major strain is physical—just finding enough energy left for three hours of education, and then drawing this out on Wednesday evenings. The paper work in between can be handled in a horizontal position as I get my quota of rest. The stress is on my physical strength, which I must not overextend.

Being able to continue professionally throughout the treatment time is my greatest blessing—eliminating whole areas of decision making and change of environment. It will make retirement at an appropriate time a manageable transition, with no regrets.

So the four CT's are interrelated harbingers of Cure!— part of the total treatment. Obviously, I am getting the best care in the world. I'm by no means completely sure I'm doing it all right! Lord, give me body wisdom extraordinaire!" [Journal entries from early February, 1983]

Chapter 8

Living With Chemotherapy - II

The progressive lymphoma had been halted, according to a chest X ray at the end of January which showed *All Clear* in the lung and along the aorta from neck to groin. The medication was holding the TB in check. But progressive weakness from the effects of the toxic drugs was a hard reality.

Would it have helped to know how such symptoms could be caused by the drugs? My oncologist would answer every question I asked, but I needed more basic information to know what questions to ask. His theory apparently is that a patient should not be warned ahead of time and, in anticipation, find symptoms that might not really be present.

It is only since starting this writing project that I have obtained helpful literature that denotes what aftereffects can be caused by specific anticancer drugs.[3] I think it would have helped me to know, because much anxiety for me centered around whether I had brought on such effects by doing too much or failing to do something necessary for good health.

If you are one who prefers not to over-anticipate bad effects from lifesaving medicines, you may want to skip this chapter. Even Vance, my companion in the well-fought fight wonders why I want to remember and rehash the critical months, now that we have lived through the worst.

38

The treatment was worse than the disease at that point in its effects on my total system and on our spirits. This was such an important period of learning, of getting in touch with inner strengths, that I reread journal entries from that time with more insight, and want the facts and feelings of that time recorded.

Chemotherapy Is No Fun!

After the first two cycles of treatment, I began experiencing leg aches. After walking four blocks one day, one knee stiffened up. Stairs began to seem like mountains. The gastrointestinal system was off kilter constantly. There were watery bags under my eyes.

Describing the big dose of Cycle #3, I reported:

> As Dr. . . . administered the vials of poison, I felt the suffusion rising in my head . . . then came the hours of restlessness, muddled thinking, not even a good high. Concentration is very fleeting and no sleep possible . . . On the dot of 6:00 p.m. the upheavals began. Every half hour there was an onslaught, a wrenching attempt to vomit up nonexistent intestinal content . . . Poor Vance almost joins the horrible chorus as he holds my head through each bout. The respites are short, then I'm at it again.

A week later came the lighter follow-up dose, and I recorded:

> There were more side effects from this dose than I've had before. Does this mean my system is debilitated from the continuing dosage? The doctor is very pleased that I'm able to keep going and says many people getting such a strong dosage are wiped out for six months, some even have to be hospitalized during treatments.
>
> He also gave me encouragement by saying that after three or four more cycles, the spacing will be two months apart. During the third phase, the dosage will be

reduced as well as the frequency of injections. Surely I
can take three or four more cycles. I have a fever blister
now, and still my puffy, watery eyes. Also a pasty color in
my face.

At this point I began a new semester of teaching an evening
college class:

My voice projected well even as I remained sitting, but I
certainly knew I was not the old peppy me . . . getting in
from the parking lot in wind and rain was probably a
foolish risk. I do not have confidence in my own
judgment about how much energy can or should be
used at one time.

Sitting here in bed, I think I have the stamina, but it
peters out quickly when I propel my body up and down
stairs. Is this feeling still related to the TB ordeal more
than the lymphoma or the treatments? None of the
doctors is helping me with that question.

How much physical effort am I capable of making? Do I
need to be more careful, or less? I am concerned about
the dizziness I have felt on several occasions. What
warning is this giving?

If the TB is controlled, can I store up some credit in the
energy bank by good rest, then draw on it for Sundays
and Wednesday nights? I am not so bankrupt as I was in
the fall, but my supply of get-up-and-go is so much less
than before I became aware of systemic illness, and I
am not yet in touch with my body wisdom.

What else is there to do but experiment, and avoid
getting caught in situations where I cannot immediately
quit and sit down. Certainly I must not try to prove how
much I can take. Patience!

No one can tell me how much to do. The doctor
seems to be egging me on, yet cautions care because
the effects of the drugs give some false signals. I am too
hyper on prednisone, then have withdrawal symptoms
when I am off it. I am not sleepy enough to get a good

nap; my muscles crave exercise. Is the chronic ache in my knee related to nerves and my inability to completely relax?"

Then came the *Valentine Day Special*, Chemotherapy Cycle #4, when:

There was an early onset of the upheavals. Actually, in the hours of waiting, when I can neither sleep, read nor think straight, I'm almost eager for the nausea to start so we can get it over with. But this was a long, hard bout, certainly a gut level response to the substance pumped into my bloodstream.

There was nothing to come up, for I'd allowed myself only a few sips of water all day . . . . Contorting spasms came almost every 15 minutes with Vance sitting close for support, his tummy rumbling in empathy!

By late in the evening my tiredness is overwhelming; I flop back on the pillow exhausted after each earthquake. This one was the worst so far, and there seems no rational way to be prepared for the gut twisting. That's what Dr. G. was hinting at: no avoidance of suffering.

Yet there's some humor in it. By about 1:30 A.M. there seemed to be longer intervals between bouts and Vance went to his bed and promptly had a dream that we had another child! These must have seemed like labor pains to him. My present pains are higher up, involving my whole system.

It was almost 5:00 A.M. before I could be about dreaming and finally came an hour of good sleep, and then another. So began the renewal process. Fortunately, the feeling of having been wrung out like a dishrag does abate and the restoration of my equilibrium does begin the day after cataclysm. The knowledge that just two more such cycles must be faced in Phase 1 is helpful. After Easter, the big blasts will be six weeks apart.

The main problem now is my extreme weakness. I took a spill at the kitchen door which is making the other knee stiff. The callouses on my feet are troublesome. Now the

*doctor asks if I have any on my hands, an expected
aftereffect of one of the drugs.*

Why could he not have mentioned that before? Soon I did
have as hard callouses on my hands as if I had been doing field
work. By March 4, "The tips of my fingers are so tender that
the most minimal tasks are made difficult, and I drop a lot of
things. Writing with pen or pencil is difficult, too. There's still
typing." But as numbness in the fingers took over, the strength
to play chords on the piano or to type dissipated:

*The extreme weakness I feel is very discouraging. To
get up on my legs from a low sitting position (like a toilet
seat) is a Herculean task. Do I need a walker?*

*My upbeat attitude is very frayed this week, and I have
to make an effort not to visualize what is ahead of us on
Monday next.*

*The ulcers in the roof of my mouth make eating
difficult, yet I know I must build up strength for the next
chemotherapy ordeal.*

*Up to now, even though the immediate aftereffects
increase in intensity and duration, I have felt somewhat
energetic in intervening days. Now I have no evidence
of improvement. Is my ambition just running too far
ahead of realistic strength?*

*The only thing keeping me going now is the flow of cards
and calls from friends and kinfolk far and near. The
hymn keeps singing in my mind, "I would be true, for
there are those who trust me . . ."*

*No one except Vance can really sense the terrible
draining of the treatments on my system, and now on my
morale. There's certainly no sense of every-day-in-
every-way-I'm-getting-better-and-better. I shall try not
to expect that. Yet, because I look fairly good out in
public, my fans are beginning to expect that.*

Here are reflections early on the morning before chemotherapy Cycle #5:

Reviewing a week when I became progressively weaker:
I used the ramp rather than the stairs to get to the second floor of the church Sunday and felt all right until 15 minutes into the sermon, when everything began to swim before my eyes. I sat, then managed a concluding sentence, and after the benediction, sat at the back to greet people.

Such weak knees, and maybe a fainter heart than before. Oh, to be able to walk confidently out of the house for a day in the woods instead of to the hematology clinic and the prospect of a day and a night in hell!

Vance came to join in the discussion with the doctor regarding the latest symptoms. I am really scared by the weakness of limbs. My pulse shows an irregular beat. The dosage may be affecting my cardiovascular system as well by now. A chest X ray is ordered, and an EKG when I come in next Monday. (The doctor can't be too alarmed if it can wait for a week.) But I am admonished to Take it Easy.

How quickly Vance left the room as the I.V. was to begin—having been sufficiently impressed by the array of vials waiting to be emptied into my poor, burning veins.

This proved to be a slightly less severe experience than the previous one. There was a longer time between each upheaval. Yet the severity of each attack was enough to make me faint, and apparently I did pass out momentarily at one point.

This is my week to empathize with handicapped persons. How to get dressed? Put on a slipover blouse so as not to have to deal with little buttons. Handicapped I certainly am by the tenderness and lack of discriminatory feeling in the tips of my fingers, but mostly by weakness in my hands, arms and legs. I cannot use scissors; putting on panty hose is a contortionist's nightmare.

Typing is easier than handwriting, but numb fingers hit wrong keys and I have to sit up in a chair to type. Perhaps too much of the prescribed bed rest is making me weaker. Why do my feet hurt as if I had been on a long hike? Just blame it on chemotherapy and don't try to figure out Why!

Don't say the English queen's visit to the U.S.A. didn't influence us. We now have a throne room—thanks to an uplifting toilet seat. I can rise gracefully again, having pulled out the towel rack from the wall in my attempts at a hoist last week.

I feel tired and weak in my knees and fingers. I really can't fix a meal in this condition. I've taken to calling Vance, "Mother"—he has to do so many little services for me. I am assured by the oncologist that this condition is not permanent. Meanwhile, I'm convinced that the troubles Job had must have been a kind of chemotherapy. What next for me?

Writing a journal entry by typewriter is not as satisfying as a leisurely stroll through these pages with pen, but I do not want to get too far behind. It helps to see the developing saga. On the whole I am in my Pollyanna phase despite more physical disability.

A week later, this report:

My weakened right hand is almost useless. The EKG showed an extra pacemaker effect in one ventricle of the heart. I started taking Lanoxin, and I'm to have no caffeine. The numbness in my fingertips means I've lost control of little things. Getting up even the three steps at our kitchen door is a big effort. I've started using a four-footed cane. Typing is next to impossible. The oncologist decided to give me an extra week between treatments because of my low blood count and weakness. He suggests these crippling effects will not go away until after Cycle #6 is out of the way. Nine months now of semi-invalidism, and I'm getting more disabled rather than less.

There is a long dry spell in the journal after that, because writing was so difficult. I started to work from an outline in preaching rather than from a carefully written script—as had been my custom.

The day after Easter I remember walking very precariously and very reluctantly to the car as if to the guillotine, on the way to Cycle #6. Why would any sane person willingly submit oneself to be poisoned? The reactions to that dosage began mid-afternoon, and I blacked out several times during the night.

One upsetting experience occurred when I tried to step up over the curb. Even with the help of the cane, my knees could not hold me up and I took a hard fall back into the street on my head. Finally I managed to get seated on the curb, made some quip about taking my ministry into the street, then crawled back to the open door of the car to maneuver myself into the seat. What a scary warning that was that I must avoid falling again.

I began sitting on a kitchen stool by the pulpit, rather than standing to preach. The feeling in my fingers and toes had not come back.

So, in the first phase, six big treatments and six small treatments in three and a half months, what had I learned?

• The humility of having to be very dependent on someone else. How do people who live alone manage during chemotherapy like mine?

• Ways of adjusting to a lot of handicaps and disabilities.

• Tenacity in the face of adversity! I'd been working on that learning for my whole life, and this was the big test.

It would have been hard to convince me during this period that "chemotherapy is your friend" for all of the troubles seemed related to the toxic drugs. The aftereffects for the immediate hours following the intravenous injections were horrid but bearable, especially as I learned to crawl back to near normalcy fairly quickly. But the overall effects of weakness and disability filled me with apprehension. For how long would I be getting worse and worse? All of these problems came from the drugs, not directly from the disease! Things were certainly not going better with chemistry.

I had reached *The Pits.* I had withstood the worst of the side effects during the first third of the treatments. With longer intervals between treatments, my body could repair and there would be more fairly good days.

Compared to the first six cycles, everything thereafter has been less wearisome and worrisome. But these days must be remembered, so that such comparisons can be savored. I was learning how to survive a sanity-threatening treatment for a life-threatening disease.

Chapter 9

Prayer and Healing

Creating meaning of the events in one's life is, of course, my life's work. Much of the work of ministry is helping people in this process, reaching for the resources for a faith journey within a community of believers.

As a "wounded healer" I could share my own experiences of the efficacy of prayer and hopefulness in a deeper way than ever before. But while I was in a sense a professional pray-er, and had cultivated skills of intercessory prayer over the years, it did not follow that I knew how to pray for myself, at least in the area of healing.

One early journal entry confesses this:

> How touched I am by some of the notes from loved ones! Being prayed for is a tangible experience. Indeed, if for brief moments I am unable to do my own praying it will be OK. I'll be upheld by the prayers of others.
>
> I remember reading that a liberal is one who works for the liberation of others, while a radical is one who works for her own liberation. It's radical prayer I must now learn—how to pray for my own healing and not worry about being selfish; how to give up being too Spartan and allow myself some coddling without feeling guilty.

Never had I been more conscious of being upheld by the Everlasting Arms, and it was God's love I felt through the tangible messages of love from the network of the caring. "The Mylanta of the spirit, coating my inner being—a cushion for the rough hours of reaction to the drugs," was one way of describing the support of all those who were praying for me. I was especially humbled by the testimony of a friend, some 20 years my senior, that her own prayer life had deepened as she prayed for me each day.

A colleague at the college asked me quite directly, "*Do you believe in divine healing?*" This is one of those questions which must be invited in for a long sojourn of contemplation and honest response.

In intercessory prayer I sincerely assume that to lift up before God any situation puts that person in the zone of healing energy. When a group of people focus on a particular person's special needs, perhaps actively praying at a particular time on a particular day, there is the possibility of psychic power being released, even when the one being prayed for does not know of the prayer conspiracy.

To be told that such prayer power is being practiced in your behalf is a humbling experience, mocking your own dubious faith. I did not know the content of such prayers, but accepted gratefully the knowledge of concern that involved so much commitment of time and energy. This may be the way God could answer my own prayers, providing channels of healing grace through the prayers of others.

A lifelong pattern of practicing the presence of God has been intensified in this crisis situation. With so much time spent physically immobile over a span of months, I had been almost literally in prayer without ceasing. The inner dialogue and hard meditation about specific needs and wider concerns was daily exercise. Letting the faces of friends flash through my mind, as I willed them into God's presence, too, sending my love to them over the thought waves, was part of my prayer life. But was I praying for my own healing?

"Do you believe in divine healing?" Isn't all healing divine? The remarkable abilities of the body and its interdependent functions—the give-and-take between this living machine and its complex mind—constitute evidence of a divine source at the heart of creation which is on the side of healing, seeking homeostasis, equilibrium and harmony.

But I do not believe in magic. I do not believe that the Creator of an ordered world makes exceptions to the laws of cause and effect for the sake of one transitory life. The miracle of healing, which can change the dynamics of any situation, often beyond scientific expectation or explanation, does not guarantee that a particular person's disease will be permanently cured, or that life will go on forever.

I was looking for no special dispensation, "no dream, no prophet ecstasies, no sudden rending of the veil of clay, no angel visitants, no opening skies." But the hymn writer's prayer was also mine: "Lord, take the dimness of my soul away."

My prayer life intensified through this experience, yet the content of my prayers continued in a familiar pattern:

• Thanks be to God for unspeakable gifts which can be cataloged and celebrated.

• "Thou, O Lord, knowest all my needs before I can even sense them."

• My faith that basic needs would be met was reinforced with each day's experience.

• I kept on praying for strength to endure; wisdom to understand how I can cooperate with the healing forces; patience and empathy for those whose lives are tortured by my tortures; overflowing love for the medical team, the researchers, the ones near and dear to me whose prayers are made in my behalf.

These were just small efforts toward praying for my own healing. It was the best I knew how to do.

I was interested in the account of Kathryn Koob, among the captured members of the U.S. Embassy staff held hostage in Iran in 1980. Reliance on the Bible, on religious hymns and scripture lessons from her youth she credited with helping her endure those days of captivity with the uncertain outcome.

"The actions I took during those 444 days," she reports in *Guest of the Revolution*[4], "were identical to those that anyone who had been raised in the Christian faith used every day to meet any crisis."

That is essentially my testimony, too. The wellsprings of faith and prayer and inspirational hymns that had brought me thus far through life were there to be tapped in the cancer crisis. I had the added advantage of a sermon and a pastoral prayer to be prepared each week, where my spiritual pilgrimage could be shared, thus enhancing the treasures to the mediator and communicator.

Kathryn Koob developed a ritualized schedule of intercessory prayer: "Mondays were days of prayer for all the institutions of the churches. Tuesday, I prayed for all the various human crises in the world: for world hunger, for those who are oppressed, for those who are ill, and for all sorts of social needs. On Wednesday I prayed for my family and my friends, starting in one corner of the U.S. and praying through all the different locations across the country."

I cannot claim such a disciplined approach. For a body undergoing chemotherapy, discipline is a problem. But I can fully understand how she turned to intercessory prayer to help get her through her own crisis. I, too, was reaching out in my prayers more extensively and intensively, focusing on the special needs of particular people.

Koob learned to pray for her captors and put her fate in God's hands. Never did I doubt that my fate, too, was in God's hands. To pray in the midst of daily changes, "O Thou who changest not, abide with me," is both prayer and affirmation. To ask for enablement to meet any experience is to have prayer answered in the asking.

However, I was not yet comfortable about specific prayers for my own healing. I didn't know how to do that! It is an area of continued exploration and learning.

Chapter 10

Living With Chemotherapy - III

Cycle #6 had marked a turning point. There would now be two months between major injections, a longer time for the cell repair work to take place. Crippling side effects lingered, with nagging problems, such as shingles, occurring frequently. Chronic illness is a drag.

There was a long time between journal entries because of paralyzed fingers. I couldn't even turn on a lamp. Walking was hazardous. I could get up easily only from the height of the bed, tolerably well from the raised toilet seat and from the back seat of the car more easily than from the front bucket seat. Of course, I had not driven the car for months.

It often seemed I was losing ground. I used a four-footed cane like a pet on a leash. The treatments, though less frequent, were just as difficult to endure as before.

Yet the second six month phase of chemotherapy provided many strokes—personally and professionally. The college where I had served as campus minister and continued as part-time instructor named me for the year's Humanitarian Award.

I had a good cry over that, hoping they were not feeling sorry for me in my present condition, nor assuming I might not be around long. Being carted out to the graduation exercises on the playing field by the campus police and making my precarious way to the podium to a standing ovation was a highlight of my life. Perhaps if I had not become a cancer patient, no one would have thought of so honoring me!

We were leading a full life, and at a Chinese restaurant I found in my fortune cookie this good omen: *You will soon recover valuables thought lost.*

The lost valuables I wanted back right then were the use of fingers and toes. A year had now passed since the first hospital diagnostic experience. I was finished with all the pills aimed at curing tuberculosis. My system could give up those antibiotics. I thought I felt better because of that.

The chronic nature of semi-invalidism is a drag. I was still largely an invalid—what a particularly unfortunate word that is in our language. How it compounds one's identity problems throughout illness. To be judged "in-valid" certainly adds insult to injury.

How comforting, then, to be so upheld by friends and family still. I had anticipated that our health crisis would be old news by now and we should not expect so much attention. Yet each week brought fresh surprises, bringing us in touch with the sorrows and joys of others and their care for us.

We Can Do

And then we heard about a We Can Do group at our hospital, and became part of this weekly circle of fellow travelers through the paths of cancer and other chronic illness. This is a national organization founded by survivors of cancer. Norman Cousins[5] is chairperson of its board of directors. Each meeting "combines presentation of educational information, use of relaxation techniques, support group strategies, and discussions and demonstration of other methods of coping."

The group we joined was co-led by the hospital social worker and a warm and competent volunteer counselor whose specialty was leading us through imagery about the locus of our disease, the role of the treatments, and the hoped-for outcome.

These exercises, based on the Simontons' work, we were encouraged to do for ourselves three times a day. I certainly did not manage that. I did begin to develop some skill in such visualization of the workings of this chemical plant that my body had become. It was like doing inner aerobics.

I therefore had more command of true relaxation as I faced Cycle #9 treatment. The expected aftereffects were weathered, and we could rejoice that the chemotherapy program was half finished.

The best part of the We Can Do group for the two of us was the new circle of friends not connected in any way with our professional lives. Hearing the stories, particularly of those who had been cancer patients for as long as ten years, gave us new perspective on our own.

It was a safe place to let down one's hair, or if you had no hair, a place to risk going without one's wig! (I had progressed from egghead at Easter to "new wave" by Veterans' Day, with eyebrows and eyelashes returning.)

We could express things at group meetings which we had not even shared with each other at home, and often gained insights on the spot about our true feelings, about patterns of response that were proving either self-defeating or somewhat effective. Always we were reinforced in our struggle toward health and wholeness regardless of the situation of the moment.

The members of the support group began to care for each other, intentionally keeping one or another in our thoughts on treatment days especially. There was a tangible mutuality without any obligation for socializing beyond our meeting day.

Our family doctor had commented that "unfortunately, the people who really need such groups are not the ones who participate." He is mistaken. Everyone needs such a support group experience through various times in life. We are grateful to have stumbled onto this one. But even they were having a hard time convincing me that "chemotherapy is your friend."

Appropriately enough, it was on Veterans' Day that I went for the Cycle #10 ordeal. After this there would be not only the longer spacing between injections, but a gradual reduction in the number and strength of the drugs administered.

We wrote to friends: "It's easier to feel hopeful when you're feeling good. But how impatiently we long to be *all better*. We marvel that you haven't tired of hearing our news by now. We are amazed and humbled by your continued prayers and love therapy. Hang in there! That's what we intend to do!"

How The Fortune Cookies Crumble

Then, on the first anniversary of our receiving the cancer diagnosis, we went with friends to the Chinese restaurant again, and this time Vance and I received *twin* fortunes: *Life for you is a dashing and bold adventure*. What a confirmation of our affirmations!

In my journal I recalled events and feelings of one year ago, when I could not have predicted celebrating another Christmas:

> There were so many unknowns, the holidays took on a special intensity then. This year, I'm overwhelmed with gratitude, feeling so close to a whole world of people. I'm a long way from normal functioning—walk so slowly, still very dependent. Yet as we shared at We Can Do this week, I found myself voicing that if it has to be, I could live on productively with present disabilities. Not that I want to!
>
> We are able to go and do, but after a few hours my head craves a pillow and a stretch-out is welcome. There is still no reserve energy, and without my wig or a jaunty scarf, the image my mirror gives back shows ravages of this year of stress and distress.

Does the fortune cookie know something my doctors don't? *"You will recover . . ."* No one promises that! CURB not CURE is their prognosis. *"Valuables thought lost?"* The treasured valuables are rediscovery of friendships old and new.

We have tapped hidden sources of stamina and strength to live through the chemotherapy so far. The oncologist gave us assurance that as soon as certain drugs are dropped from the repertoire in these final months, the nerve functions in my fingers and toes will be restored.

Assuredly, life is a bold and dashing adventure, even for a semi-invalid cancer patient who has survived another year. I tied a red paper poinsettia to the four-footed cane for the holiday season.

Chapter 11

Visualization as "Adjuvant" Therapy

Is Cancer the Enemy?

Obviously the chemotherapy treatments were keeping me alive as well as keeping me disabled. Had this love-hate relationship with chemotherapy kept me from coming to terms with cancer itself?

A prominent TV evangelist announced a special vision in which Jesus Christ informed him that cancer is the work of the Devil and must be fought as in a righteous war.

I reasoned, however, that those cancer cells—confused, weak, disorganized and a consummate threat to the body's health—are still one's own cells, not aliens such as bacteria. They are produced within one's own body as a natural outcome of cause and effect, only partially understood as yet by scientists.

But they are there with the Creator's permission, as it were. If "a weed is just a plant in the wrong place," can the cancer cells be seen in a similar light? They are indeed misplaced as well as misinformed, but essentially neutral as they get started.

True, they can become invasive of other tissues and organs. If one's immune system is deficient and fails to recognize the misplaced cells and fails to destroy them before runaway growth takes over, they will crowd out healthy cells to cause disorder, disease, death.

Most suggested visualization of cancer treatment is that of an all-out war waged against the wrongly programmed cancer cells. If not actually an invader to start with, cancer is seen as an aberration caused by various factors that are enemies of health. To cure cancer, these enemies must be sought out, destroyed, removed, excised, and/or bombarded with chemicals or radiation X rays.

There is general agreement that a patient's attitudes can help the immune system cooperate in these counterattacks against the cancer cells. One is encouraged to visualize the immune system cells as more numerous and more powerful than those causing disease, and the treatment as much more potent still, affecting the normal cells in the process, but not harming them beyond repair.

A certain chemical shot into the patient's bloodstream releases an array of complex molecules to fight a specialized part of the battle. One drug can interrupt the growth process and paralyze some cells in mid-division. Another one sneaks inside the cancer cells, stopping them from making the genetic material they need to reproduce. One, shaped like a vitamin that the voracious cell needs, is quickly gobbled up. Once inside, the molecule proves as indigestible as a grain of sand, so the cell chokes and dies. Under a multiple-chemical onslaught, the tumor cells falter, stop, retreat, leaving millions of their dead behind.

These become suggested images for visualizing the power of the treatment. Accepting this Armageddon model, some people visualize shooting matches or chemical warfare going on inside their bodies.

The military imagery was incompatible with my belief system, and I began playing with more domestic scenes. I could see the cancer cells as small black ants, swarming over the kitchen sink, their ranks swelling with no end in sight. There is nothing I hate worse than to wake up to such a kitchen scene, so those ants were quite detestable. I had a strong urge to get rid of them pronto.

The toxic drugs injected through my veins could act as powerful DDT to stop those no-good creatures in their tracks. Perhaps a spray gun is just as violent an instrument as a machine gun or flame thrower, but I could accept that!

Our We Can Do counselor cautioned, however, that to think of cancer cells as hard and black like ants might prove a negative image, that I should try for something not alive and of a nothing color—something soft that can be broken down, disintegrated then flushed away. Those cancer cells are alive, I reasoned, growing and reproducing beyond reason.

As I experimented with other symbols, I found I could deal with a fungus-type growth appearing and spreading around the edges of other functioning tissue clumps. Then I could see the powerful white blood cells as a corps of sanitation workers (such as those who nightly scrub down the sidewalks in China's cities while the populace sleeps, leaving places clean beyond belief as morning breaks!). Dressed in white, and with small miners' lights on their foreheads, these efficient workers are on a constant search and destroy mission to spot any creeping tentacles of mold or fungi. This imagery began to work for me.

Far from seeing cancer as an archenemy to be met by the overkill of machine guns, I even visualized at one time later when the drug portions of my treatment had been considerably reduced, that the recurring proliferation of the cancer cells might be as benign as cotton candy! Spun sugar, which rapidly expands in volume to take up a lot of space without substance, when left to sit in pure air disintegrates rapidly into a little sticky mess, easily rinsed away. Could the immune system corps of sanitation engineers use atomizers to reduce the flimsy cancer cells to such rubble?

I was interested in reading an account of Henry Weaver's *Confronting the Big C*[6] to find that he also had to substitute other images for the military models most self-help programs suggest.

Perhaps we are both rationalizing when we reject the bad guy/ good guy images. Yet could it be that answer is merely one dramatic symptom, out of many of ultimately self-destructive tendencies upon which our modern civilization is based? Must every struggle, both within and without, be a matter of dividing good from bad, friend from enemy, health from illness?

Taking seriously the ecology of both outer and inner environment, will we look at all conflicts of our life in a different way? Perhaps no enemy really exists. Do all factors proceed in a harmonious manner, coexisting and supporting each other?

Even cancer may be a natural adjustment of the body to the accumulation of toxins ingested and accumulated through years of eating unnatural diets, breathing in carcinogens, living in artificial environments. Even misconceptions and ultimately self-destructive tendencies of striving, competition, divisiveness on which society operates play a part in inner ecological imbalance.

Michio Kushi makes some of these points in his book, *The Cancer Prevention Diet.*[7] I was not persuaded that his macrobiotic diet is the ultimate answer, certainly not persuaded to switch that dramatically while in the midst of chemotherapy. His underlying philosophhy of life, however, contains much food for thought. He believes that cancer is a product of our own daily behavior, including our thinking, our life-style and our daily way of eating. The cell is only the terminal of a long organic process, not a phenomenon isolated from its surroundings and other body functions.

It is the degenerative diseases, including cancer, which have dramatically increased in recent years as the ultimate cause of death. Kushi believes that we will all be affected by such diseases, especially in highly technological societies, until a new, peaceful way of life is established in place of our present frenzy.

If we can learn to deal with cancer not as an enemy, but as the body's last drastic effort to prolong life, we may dare to hope for a lasting solution to the multiple ills of society itself just over the horizon! This is holistic thinking par excellence.

In Kushi's book are hints for creative imagery along the lines of cooperation within the natural environment, aimed at overcoming egocentric views, and moving toward more universal concerns. Self-reflection involving our higher consciousness would lead one to observe, review, examine and judge thoughts and behavior in a context of the larger order of nature—what might be called the law of God. One paragraph in particular speaks to me:

> *By appreciating the gift of life in all its manifestations, we increase the universe's faith in us, and life becomes an endlessly amusing and joyful adventure. If we have cancer, e.g., we accept what it has to teach us about ourselves. We never lament over our fate and blame it on an accident, karma, evil spirits, or an indifferent cosmos. We look for a source of our problems from within ourselves, and when we make a mistake, we learn from it and gratefully move on.*

Is cancer the enemy? It was simple to say, when someone asked why I use a cane, "I'm fighting cancer."

After reading Kushi's words, I wanted to keep faith with the universe's faith in me. The warrior image did not fit. Codefendant of the healing energies, cheerleader for the body's immune system, inner ecology engineer—something along these lines was called for to replace the pugnacious imagery which could in turn affect attitude.

Visualization and Prayer

The self-reflection that comes with a disciplined plan of visualization qualifies, I believe, as a kind of praying. One way to define prayer is "paying attention". One consciously prepares a receptive, informed, not-too-impatient mental and spiritual environment and then focuses petition on a given concern.

Prayer or visualization directed toward the healing of disease would put one in harmony with rather than at war with biochemical realities. The first step is a focus on breathing more deeply and rhythmically, paying attention to this central fact of continued exsitence. With tension reduced, step two can be taken: picture in your mind a tranuquil scene, familiar or idealized, to which you can return at will for total immersion in peace and joy, your own private heaven. (Think how often we allow ourselves sleepless nights conjuring up our own private hells, worrying about what might happen to ourselves or loved ones.)

It is recommended that one practice such exercises three times a day. I didn't even strive for that. Even to hold myself to a once-a-day practice of visualization would have added stress to a schedule crowded with the deadlines for ingesting numerous prescription drugs.

Yet I did not rely on times of panic or when the spirit moved me to do the exercises learned at our weekly group session. About three times a week I listened to tapes or reviewed the step-by-step pattern. The breathing exercises I used more frequently. I am able now to enter into satisfying visualization experience at will.

As with the practice of prayer, the "Practice of the Presence of God" that develops through disciplined prayer experiences at certain times in one's life, techniques once learned do not disappear, even if we neglect the use of those muscles from time to time. This is not to argue against regular, daily devotional exercises. It is just to be honest about my own life pattern, sick or well, and to be glad for the resources I can tap into when needed.

· "Oh, what peace we often forfeit, oh, what needless pain we bear, all because we do not carry everything to God in prayer," the old hymn from childhood reminds us. In a similar way, we forfeit the benefits of intentional visualization as a pause that refreshes, that heightens awareness of body needs, emotions, spiritual responsibility.

It is available to anyone, anywhere, whenever needed. It requires no prescription given or to be refilled, no insurance forms for reporting. It is the one area where a patient does not have to rely on any other person. Regardless of disability or dependency, it is true do-it-yourself therapy. It does require energy and purposiveness, and being led through the process by a competent counselor is a great bonus.

I have called such visualization adjuvant therapy—never a substitute for medical attention and treatment, nor ever in conflict with medical procedures or prescriptions.

So far as I can see, visualization of this sort is at no point in conflict with anyone's belief system. It is not a replacement for religious devotion and practice. The content of the imagery will be influenced by one's faith experience and religious vocabulary. For me, adding symbols from my faith heritage— Biblical images, and especially phrases from hymns which continue to sing their way through my memory—tends to enhance and make more vivid the visualization experience.

My prayer life has become more healing-oriented. With more sense of intention, I push to the deepest levels of understanding God's will. I focus on marshalling the divine energies, willing them to course through my cells, my system, my decision making, my relationships with new intensity.

Spiritual health or a balanced inner ecology, call it either one. The answer to such prayer includes acceptance of what must be and a willingness to be a ready participant in the healing process insofar as I am given understanding of it. Prayer is keeping open those energy channels.

Visualization is also a kind of dramatic play for adults. The young child manipulates toys or household objects, imaginatively creating a setting and a rudimentary plot for invented characters. Oblivious to those around her, a three year old can sustain interest in such activity for a long time. Make-believe is a way of handling the confusions and stresses of being little and powerless. She is at least the equal of those toy playmates and master of their environment.

As grown-ups we have the capacity for abstractions. Then why check ourselves out of such dramatic play with ideas and fantasies? Why not enjoy such imagined places of beauty and calmness, such sights and sounds and smells and textures? This is the stuff of poetry!

With a jolt, I realized that all during the severity of illness and treatments, I had written no poetry. In other crisis periods of life, poetry therapy has been an important coping activity for me, no matter how crowded the agenda of my life just then. Yet during long months of enforced idleness, only an occasional notation in my journal had the ring of poetry to it.

My sense of humor was operating at full steam. Why no poetry writing? Is it indeed one-tenth inspiration, nine-tenths perspiration? I had been too sick, too weak, to muster energy to translate feelings into the rhythm and rhymes of poems, even with all that time for meditation and meaning search during the long and grueling chemotherapy treatment months.

To be fair to my creative muse, I had written a sermon each week, and was told by at least one parishioner, "We are certainly not being cheated by your illness." Chemotherapy takes its pound of flesh and of mental energy. There was nothing left over for poetry writing.

I do testify that the visualization exercises released some of the play instinct, and as I recover strength, perhaps the poetry will flow again. Play and prayer and poetry are agents of healing and wholeness, along with humor.

In Pursuit of the Hi-Pro Glow

Another part of the visualization program which we practiced at group meetings, and at home, was to picture one's ideal self. In this you must picture yourself as you would like to be: healthy, vital, energetic. This is the image of the hoped-for outcome of treatment, both medical and psychological.

The ideal image I carry with me comes from a televised commercial for a certain dog food. In it the family pet is seen capering happily within a complete circle of light, positively scintillating in the "hi-pro glow of good health." That's what I want for myself. How I long for that sense of well-being and vigor, that ability to move my body through space. Oh, to have that kind of bouncing energy and high jumping capacity!

To be truly healthy again, I would radiate the inner light that is part of my experience, at least sporadically, so that an outer glow like that around the TV canine would replace the anemic look my mirror gives back now. I'd be walking with the old clip in my step, instead of being shaky and tentative, reaching for support. The hi-pro glow is certainly my goal, and the circle of light seems real enough to touch. It gives off waves of energy even as I think about it!

Light is an effective symbol in many ways. One can imagine laser beams shrinking the tumor, first by exposing the cancer cells as imposters, then stopping their reproductive capacities. I have not received radiation X rays, yet I sometimes feel that the chemicals given to me act in such a way.

One thinks, too, of the healthy process of photosynthesis, sunlight acting on plants to produce what plant cells need to grow. Could letting in more light encourage the immune system to more efficiency?

There are theological implications of light. We need the light of knowledge about what is really happening in our bodies, and the light of knowledge of the unconditional love of God. Light carries a sense of cleansing power, illuminating dark places we cannot easily see, helping us to be aware of unhealthful attitudes as well as cancerous cells in tissues. Light spells a warmth that is comforting and healing, relaxing stress and distress.

One of the visualization exercises offered by our counselor I especially appreciated is called "the golden bubble of light." Her taped message takes one through half an hour of letting the part of the mind that makes pictures put you in a bubble of yellow light, the color of the sun, the color of infinity. Almost like a mantra, one repeats, "I am in a bubble of light and only light can come to me and only light can be here," and then taking this light consciously into various parts of the body, into the bone marrow itself, into each cell and capillary of the blood stream in your imagining, strengthening the sense of the immune system and overwhelming any problems of disease or of fear.

To live and function within such a pervasive environment of light is a good goal for anyone. This puts the emphasis on living life fully at any moment, with less concern about how many moments stretch ahead. It offers an inner well-being now regardless of that elusive concept—cure.

All this visualization was well and good between chemo-therapy treatments. Intellectually I had come a long way from the bitterness felt by many cancer patients about the diabolical treatments which either "disfigure, burn or poison" the body. The end of a long program of treatments was in sight. I could hope for the ideal of the bubble of light existence. Even though the toxins were the villains accounting for a lot of discomforts and disorder in my system, I could almost call chemotherapy friend rather than foe and assume that the road to recovery would be found on the map of our future. Even if I might never move along that road as fast as I wished, I might recover the hi-pro glow of good health.

I tried visualizing what it would be like to drive the car again or to play tennis. As I mentally went through each necessary sequential motion, my muscles began to wake up and want very much to respond. The nice part about playing tennis in this way is that you can visualize returning all the balls with brilliant strategy, and you can win all the points!

Chapter 12

One Finish Line Is Crossed

With the turn of a New Year, there were three more cycles of treatment to face in a six-month period which, under the best of circumstances, would have tried stamina as well as soul.

A big change in life-style was scheduled for the end of June, when with birthday #65 I could retire with dignity and pension. But leaving this pastorate meant leaving the parsonage where we had lived for five years.

The search for a home for retirement years in the same general area provided some fun. We looked at a number of houses, trying to visualize what our life might be like in each possible new environment and finally we found a house to buy which seemed to fit.

My physical handicaps and weakness did not augur well for the rigors of getting moved. Stooping over was treacherous and tiring, stretching next to impossible. Cleaning out a closet for half an hour put me horizontal for the next three. I tried not to think ahead to the moving which had to be accomplished by July 1st.

There was certainly enough else to occupy mind and muscles in the busy professional life that spring. Two cancer patients among my parishioners, both age 90, completed the cycle of their lives during those months, one in a home hospice situation which was a wonderful experience to share. Somehow

I got myself up a steep flight of stairs to visit her week by week, to be inspired by her alert and faith-filled approach to the progression of the terminal disease. Those two memorial services took on special meaning for me.

I had gained strength and mobility with the spacing out of treatments and reduction of dosage. I could walk—really walk—four blocks at a time, before Cycle #12 in early March sent the blood count plunging again.

It would take at least a month more for my body to deal with that dosage of drugs in characteristic fashion. Familiar side effects would crimp my ambitiousness and my walking ability, but I would not report to the oncologist for three months. So the March 11 final injection seemed like graduation day.

Everyone around me caught the spirit of our having fought the good fight, run the race, finished the course. One friend brought over a bottle of champagne, but I hesitated mixing alcohol with all those other chemicals in my system. On Sunday, two lay leaders of the church surprised me at the announcement time with presentation of a Certificate of Completion, and in response I dramatically ripped off the most recent bandaids covering my needle marks, creating a new ritual—like the burning of a mortgage.

Did I really think I was at the end of all treatment for lymphoma? I certainly felt a great sense of relief, and some pride, that we had weathered the slings and arrows of those 16 months. Both of us let down a little, only to discover how truly tired we were after this ordeal which had lasted from December 1982 to March 1984. What an enormous amount of energy we had expended to keep on keeping on.

The Journal records:

I can't seem to get enough rest. I caught a cold from Vance which was quickly controlled by antibiotics, however. Then bloodshot eyes sent me to our doctor for special drops. The frustrations of closing escrow were trying; getting our things sorted for discarding and packing was a very tiring, little-by-little occupation. I just keep hoping for endurance to accomplish the big move.

We continued to receive strokes from former colleagues as they included us in activities of interest. I was asked to participate in a creative learning experience at one of the colleges. It meant sitting on a folding chair for three hours of afternoon time when I would normally have been resting horizontally. I was able to make my way up the steps to the podium for my part in the program.

The exhiliration of seeing old friends and doing my thing in the old pattern certainly buoyed me up. It was quite a test of stamina, of course, and it triggered a night of chilling nightmares.

The Nightmare Lingers On

I have not yet mentioned the recurring pattern of vicious nightmares—the subconscious mind's way of registering the horror of being periodically poisoned by toxic drugs.

Usually I dreamt that wild animals were attacking me. I would not come fully awake before being painfully gripped on arm or leg by savage teeth. (One of the body's reactions to the drugs which affect nerve functions has been a lot of cramping of muscles, especially in bed.)

The dream late in April involved being held by terrorists in a building where every promising escape route would lead only to a precipitous edge as the descending stairs would end abruptly. A little girl (the child in me?) showed me the way out, but would not let me take a cookie off a plate near the exit! Finally I did walk out only to find another dead-end stairway. Then I spied an unimpeded access across a wide street into a big convention hall where colleagues from various past connections greeted me warmly. I made my way toward the platform and spotted my husband's bald spot in a front row seat. He didn't seem especially glad to see me.

Did I wake up quickly at that point! It was better not to spend too much time analyzing that one.

More recently I've had dreams about leaving my cane behind or forgetting to take it when I leave the house. Interestingly enough, though I've used a cane for a year and a

half, we have not yet stopped at the Department of Motor
Vehicles to ask for a permit card for using parking places for
the handicapped. Deep down we have viewed these handicaps
of mine as a temporary condition, related to the treatment
more than to the disease—assuming all functions would return
once I am finished with chemotherapy.

And now, we asked ourselves: Had we really finished the
course? If so, did it mean the commencement of a recovery
program? Was I all well now, since the oncologist had
essentially discharged me, wanting only to monitor my
progress in periodic checkups?

We still felt the need for the We Can Do discussions and
exercises as we waited to see what would happen next. It was
great now to feel the wind in my own hair, but I was not yet
having smooth sailing—either internally or in my locomotion.
Just where was I as a cancer patient? Free of intravenous
injections for three months, but how about "free at last"? Were
we waiting for another shoe to drop?

We did not have a long wait.

Tricky Diagnosis Again

One night I casually rubbed my hand across the mostly
unfeeling toes, and was surprised to have pus burst out from
one, where an ingrowing nail had triggered an infection.
Because of the numbness, I had had no pain sensations and still
have no idea how long it had been building up.

It took a week of home remedies to clear it up. How
vulnerable one can be with frozen toes. Then I discovered two
swelling lymph nodes in the right groin. Again, it was an
accidental discovery, since I do not do a daily body check.
Besides, they did not hurt.

"Will they just go away? Of course not!" I confided to my
journal. I decided not to be coy about it and told family
members about them—but held off consulting a doctor for
several reasons. Mainly, we had to get that move accomplished
before I might be grounded again. (How little I had learned
about seeking help for symptoms I could not readily explain to

myself—or about how life managed to go on even when I'm not involved in and responsible for everything!)

The question was: Which doctor should I call? Somehow we managed the move to the new house. Two days later I saw our family physician who could not believe that lymphoma was the cause of those localized lumps. If the lymphoma were active (again), swollen nodes should have popped up throughout the whole system. Perhaps it was an infection of some sort—considering the infected toe was also on the right side. No fever, no pain—one learns to value such ordinary symptoms as aids to diagnosis. Dr. M. thought I could wait until the scheduled appointment with the oncologist three weeks hence to have these new nodes checked out.

A week later, however, the enlarging nodes were giving me pain and made walking difficult. I took my lumpy self back to the hematology clinic two weeks early. The oncologist, too, was perplexed. Any problem should be system wide rather than be so localized. He tended to agree with Dr. M. about inflammation of some sort.

"Don't panic," said the disappointed doctor. "There are several combinations of drugs we can use. We still have a lot of options, if it's just lymphoma."

Imagine talking about "just lymphoma"!

Then on June 1st, the day my Medicare card became operative, he sent me to use it at the outpatient department of the hospital for an ultrasound test. The doctor seemed panicky because of the swollen veins in the upper leg.

Phlebitis was ruled out by the interesting tests in the nuclear medicine lab, but I was put back on prednisone again. This kept me going through the rest of that month, through the retirement day festivities.

It was now three and a half months since "finishing the course" of chemotherapy treatments. More than two months had gone by in getting a diagnosis for a new, though related, problem of localized lymph node swelling and irritation of the veins.

A postgraduate course was in the offing!

Chapter 13

Chemotherapy Revisited

Checking into the hospital again had its humorous moments! We were asked to sign the usual permission forms and Vance noticed the description of the operation as typed in by a perhaps sleepy intake clerk: "Resection of two lymph nodes in the right *growing* area."

Hereafter in our family we spoke not only about a "pain in the neck" but about pains in the growing area as symbolic of a variety of frustrations, not always resectable!

Our memo to friends in late July 1984 describes the next phase of the chemotherapy career, from which we hoped we had retired.

> On July 3 biopsy surgery resected two swollen lymph nodes in the right groin, first detected early in May.... These show Progressive Lymphoma, Stage 4—the same diagnosis as that in December 1982.
>
> My oncologist interprets that as "the lymphoma came back"—localized in the nodes and veins just below the groin in the right leg.
>
> On July 10 a new combination of drugs was injected—needles and nausea again and many of the same aftereffects in the system (I may even lose the hair recently restored), but on a smaller scale, and on a six-week schedule.

My question was, How many of these cycles will there be? The answer, Enough. How will you know when it's enough? When there is no more swelling of lymph nodes. This localization is not the textbook expectation.

Trying to cheer me up, the doctor told me of one patient who's been on a similar schedule of treatments every three months for seven years. It did not cheer me up, for the prospect of chronic treatments and less-than-good health is discouraging, especially when I have experienced some return of strength and fair walking ability. The one good factor is that I had not had to adjust to retirement, for we've been too busy with all the medical procedures in this first month.

We concluded this letter:

the drugs can keep this condition below the life threatening level. Your interaction with us makes that life worth living. Love and friendship are powerful medicine, and we'll take all we can get. Thanks!

The oncologist had assured me that any new program of chemotherapy would be less severe, in no way so destructive to my energy as in the first experience. He talked about oral drugs I had not previously been given. In wishful thinking, I had translated that into "no more intravenous."

How devastated I was to walk into the treatment room, after the biopsy had confirmed the same Stage 4 Lymphoma, to find those vials ready and waiting for me. I felt betrayed, and very sorry for myself. The next few days, I hit bottom emotionally.

But life goes on. The vacation from drugs for almost four months had allowed my system to reach a stronger status, and I now withstood the aftereffects of this program more easily. However, as we passed the second anniversary of my being a chemotherapy patient, the basic lymph node swelling had not been stopped in its tracks, and experimentation with different patterns and timing of medication kept on. At times I felt I might get the Guinea Pig of the Year award.

I began to discover that when the nodes in the groin swelled and irritated the veins in the upper leg, walking became painful—often the pain persisted through the night. Pain had not been much of a factor in the cancer experience up to now. Several nights I seriously tried to pray for specific healing, directing meditation to the more localized areas, even doing my own laying on of hands at the site of the inflammation, willing the drugs to maximum effectiveness.

My attitude toward chemotherapy had changed considerably, despite the irritations it still caused in my system—like the drying of my mouth and the cramping of my muscles. When the swelling appeared before it was time to report for the next treatment, I knew I needed my "fix" and the drugs began to seem more friend than foe.

Of course, anyone who takes aspirin is practicing chemotherapy, although the term is used most for cancer-fighting toxic chemicals. Prednisone, for example, reduces the symptoms, but also exacerbates other physical problems—such as elevating the blood sugar level. So I must take medicine to control the diabetes.

Indeed, I see the morning array of pills as a sort of orchestra, one instrument providing counterpoint to another's theme song. The internal music produced is not yet a symphony, and I know I am not the conductor! With their help, however, I keep functioning at a fair pace. But chemotherapy is no longer an arch villain, and I am more able to visualize the cancer as the culprit now that we are dealing with a local manifestation of this system-wide condition.

It's been hard to visualize as a tumor the widespread tumorous condition of the whole lymph system. There is no immediate vision of being free of it, but the medics and medicines have the upper hand. I'm making a career of cooperating with them and with all the healing energy available in being alive now.

The predictable side effects are not welcome. I still feel that I'm giving my "body to be burned" by those chemicals. The veins of my arms protest each injection and the skin burns at the needle sites, giving some idea of what is happening inside those veins throughout the body.

But to further paraphrase St. Paul, "If I have not love, it profiteth me nothing." So I accept with love the wisdom of the researchers, the skill and caring of my medical team. I am grateful to live in a part of the world where these treatments are available and well-tested, and where our health insurance allows us to afford them.

Chapter 14

Dealing with the Perceptions of Others

But You Look So Well

How often a cancer patient hears the phrase, "But you look so well!" No one minds being told that, but voice inflection may suggest that you have no right to look well and claim to be so sick! Remembering movie scenes of haggard, wasting-away bodies and Camille-like deathbed scenes, people may expect the cancer patient to be an object of pity.

Most people are but vaguely aware of how the treatment of cancer has changed in just a decade, with an emphasis now on prolonging life and improving quality of life even though cure be not guaranteed.

If one has lost a chunk of pounds over the course of illness or treatment, looking better figure-wise may be a secondary benefit—albeit a very expensive weight reduction program. Several nutritionists in my friendship circle noted that the extra weight I had carried around for so long may have helped my body to deal with the wear and tear of the drugs' side effects better than if I had been skinny when I became a chemotherapy patient.

It is nice to have my new slimness noticed. Yet the mirror reports realistically some of the ravages of two years of illness, and when the surprised reaction comes, "But you look so well!"—it is easy to feel defensive. One is tempted to put on an invalid act. You know all too well how flimsy is the stamina and you don't want your friends to expect too much of you.

The perceptions of others have a direct effect on your own self-image, your sense of identity and your will to cope creatively. I began to note the changes not only in my own perceptions but also in those around me as they dealt with my identity as a cancer patient.

It is clear that many persons feel uncomfortable if not actually threatened by contact with someone who has cancer. Co-learners in our We Can Do group report that even intimate friends may find it hard to touch or embrace them—as if fearing contagion.

A friend learned that her daughter-in-law had cautioned the children, "Stay away from Grandmother at Christmas time, because she has cancer." Cancer patients returning to the workplace after some phase of treatment, or even after being declared cured, experience job discrimination. A clergy colleague believes that he was dropped from committees in church organizations outside his own parish as soon as his unfavorable diagnosis was known.

I am blessed with a wide circle of perceptive and courageous friends, family and professional colleagues and did not experience much discomfort from the gloom and doom perceptions of others. For one thing, I usually initiate talk about cancer without euphemisms, clearing the way for callers to be less fearful of upsetting me. When told, "But you look so well," I can respond, "Thank you. Tell that to my lymph nodes."

That Little Six-Letter Word!

It may not be the four-letter words that give the most problems! One contribution the growing tribe of us who are cancer patients can make to our contemporaries may be to name the culprit, for as the very young child discovers and primitive people believe, when you can name something you have achieved a measure of control over it! Even medical professionals think up all kinds of ways to avoid using the term, cancer.

A person introduced himself to our support group as one with a "non-benign malignancy." "But I don't have cancer," he insisted at the beginning of the session. He finally learned to say the dread word in group sessions, perhaps not at home.

People may avoid cancer patients because they do not dare acknowledge the existence of such a curse. It is high time their perceptions are challenged, as roughly two-thirds of those around them experience at least a brush with this modern menace. By the year 2000 perhaps half the population will know cancer intimately.

I've enjoyed nudging some friends into honest facing of these realities by letting them know it is all right to talk about my cancer condition.

But You're So Cheerful!

Besides, I smile a lot. It is a habit I see no reason to break. But this also comes as a surprise, perhaps as an affront, to some people who cannot believe one's cheerfulness is genuine. In their perception, a cancer patient has nothing to smile about. It must be mere whistling in the dark to keep up one's spirit.

One man dropped out of our support group after three sessions, because we were not depressed enough. The good-natured bantering and sharing of jokes (as well as "organ recitals" of our current ailments) seemed inappropriate to him, coming as it did from this motley collection of cancer victims.

True, our bodies are undergoing drastic treatments. We are not what we used to be. Depression can hit any one of us at any time, sometimes induced by the medications. Tears as well as chuckles may be just under the surface—and are equally acceptable. Meanwhile, little pleasures in life's relationships and events take on added significance, especially when shared.

We can laugh at ourselves. Such laughter Norman Cousins has called "inner jogging"—a form of exercise available to even the most disabled or clumsy among us.

Ironically, a cancer patient's cheerfulness may be almost offensive to one who comes to give comfort and condolence. There are always some "Job's friends" who are sure they know what will do you good. When you speak honestly about your condition, they become uncomfortable. After all, they have come to cheer you up, to distract you from thinking about this awful cancer reality.

When I say, in a normal tone of voice, that lymphoma will be my constant companion for the foreseeable future, one friend feels that I am denying my faith. "That's no way for a Christian to talk! If you have faith, you must always expect the best!" (My perception is that a foreseeable future is the best.)

"Why put so much emphasis on the physical effects of the treatment and the disease in your reports?" another wants to know. "Why not speak only of the salutary influence of prayer and good thoughts and hopefulness?"

Probably I do not sound as pious as a preacher is expected to sound!

Still another friend worries that I shall put too much reliance on the benefits of the imagery and visualization techniques as a form of self-hypnosis. She worries that I might be tempted into self-help cures, or might give up following the doctors' orders.

These friends are telling me more about themselves than they are about me, and I love them for their concern. But I must continue to work out my own salvation, with prayer and some fasting, grateful for their honesty even as they accept mine, and humbled by their risk of involvement with me in this adventure.

This journal record and these reflections are for them and for me as participants together in a venture toward healing.

The Getting Better and Better Myth

How hard it is to give up the every-day-in-every-way-getting-better-and-better expectations about illness and medical treatments. If something ails you, go to the doctor, who cures you, or certainly makes you feel better.

Under chemotherapy, however, you go to the doctor perhaps feeling rather fit, and come out feeling worse. You face days of unpleasant aftereffects. What a lot of faith is necessary on your part and on the part of those who care about you to deal with the up-and-down nature of chronic disease with a measure of realism and hope at the same time.

The cancer patient has to help friends understand this. Some of my parishioners were as devastated as I was when I had to go back on chemotherapy after we thought the regimen was completed, or when I became lame again after having regained ability to walk four blocks just two weeks earlier. A measure of hope died.

It was I who had to comfort them in their disappointment that my progress was not a steady climb. Fortunately, there were also those in the congregation to whom chronic disease, including bouts with cancer, was no stranger. These role models continue to be important members of our support team.

It takes patience on the part of friends to sustain their care-giving to a chronic patient. The balance between positive thinking and realistic facing of circumstance is a fine line. Both are components of true hopefulness, and my friends and family and I encourage each other in the learning of patience.

Since the original manuscript for this journal was put together, I have participated in several workshops regarding ministry with those who have chronic illnesses and have included in Appendix III an outline of hints for those who call on such patients.

Perceptions of the Family Members

People began to give me more credit for courage than was warranted. Because I kept up my usual professional activities, despite difficulty with climbing stairs or use of fingers, I kept receiving compliments for bravery to the point of embarrassment.

The truth is, I could not see an alternative to just coping with each new complication, short of resigning from life altogether. I did not make a conscious choice to "have a good attitude" but it does help to have developed some psychospiritual survival strategies all along life's way. Reserve coping skills have come to my rescue in this time of extreme crisis.

Neither the coping nor the cheerfulness was accomplished alone! It was tonic for the spirit to have my closest companion express appreciation for my positive attitude. Like a self-fulfilling prophecy, Vance's expectation of my continued "good spirit" did much to keep me keeping on. It was like an unwritten mutual defense treaty between us! My overall cheerfulness was not forced, however. It welled up naturally with the tangible care and encouragement that came to us each day, along with each day's internal upsets and discomforts.

It has taken me too long to become sensitive to the effect of the long, drawn out ordeal on the key person in my support system, my ever-present spouse. At times, of course, my reliance on his care had been so complete there was no energy left to worry about how he was taking it. Compared to me, Vance has always been a stoic about his feelings. His actions bespoke unconditional love and quick attention to needs. Often he indicated that my generally positive approach to each day's adventures or misadventures helped him, too. That put off the need to deal with my guilt feelings over what my illness was doing to his freedom for retirement.

The one thing which seemed to worry Vance was that I tried to do too much, yet he did not want me to give in to the use of a wheel chair. Thus he compelled me to put forth sometimes heroic efforts to get to and fro during periods of greatest weakness.

As I gradually improve in walking skills, still needing help on steps without railings, I often see that Vance has trained himself, as the parent of a preschool child does, to automatically turn and offer a hand at the precise moment I have needed help up or down a curb! Will it be hard for him to relinquish such protective custody if I get closer to the hi-pro glow of healthy mobility and become more independent again?

The people who live with a patient are caught in a double bind between being overprotective and not protective enough. One friend reports that her husband worries if he hears her open the aspirin bottle surreptitiously to treat a headache, assuming that she is not telling him about some more troubling symptom!

Such honest communication about needs and feelings is an obligation for both patient and close care-giver. It was beneficial for us to participate together in the support group— even though some of the group did not want family members there. They felt freer to discuss pain and fears with peers and wanted to spare their family the anxiety of knowing what was really bothering them. In our case, we often revealed feelings in the group sessions we had not expressed to each other at home, sometimes discovering insights on the spot.

I keep looking for changes in my own perceptions and behavior, particularly in the area of practicing patience. Inevitably there are some changes in the relationships between the two of us in the intensified mutual dependence of patient/care-giver roles. After 35 years of marriage, there are still discoveries to be made about each other.

Our group counselor noted with amazement that we still laughed at each other's jokes! However, I came to realize that one habit of mine had become an annoyance to my closest companion: living with Pollyanna can be a pain!

A burglary occurred within the first month of the occupancy of our new home that triggered understandable anger and resentment, not only over the valuables lost but over the loss of time needed to file reports, arrange for better window security, and the like. We had been robbed of peace of mind as well. It is an outrageous experience.

Surprisingly, I had little emotional reaction to the event. Having a life-threatening disease has changed my perspective on what is worth worrying about. There just seems no time or energy to waste on impatient reaction to minor irritations and annoyances. I found myself saying even about the burglary, "It could have been worse."

That was the last straw for Vance, who could now direct some of his diffused anger and frustration at my lack of anger! With more vehemence than is characteristic of him, he sneered something about my "always putting a good face on things!"

I saw with a flash that it is not necessarily easy to live with Pollyanna, the glad girl. I also began to notice how often I resorted to the old bromide, "It could have been worse," which at that point was so irritating to my spouse!

The right to complain is a basic human right which I have always liberally exercised. It was a surprise to see Vance give in to this natural response. It also made me more aware of how much strain the illness these past couple of years has been for him—carrying as he did more than his share of the burdens during our long health crisis.

Has he changed? Have I changed? I know the experience of being a cancer patient, and especially a chemotherapy patient, has changed my perceptions about what is worth fretting about. I am amazed at my new equanimity in the face of frustrations and setbacks. If this is one component of patience, perhaps I am learning a little of it. By the same token, I wonder if Vance is learning how to express natural frustrations a little more openly than has been his wont.

The involvement of our children through these intense two years has been an important component of our experience, even though they no longer reside under our roof. To say that I rely on each of them is an understatement. There are certain things only a daughter can do for a mother!

The son who lives furthest away underwent two serious bouts with illness during these same two years. How we longed to be at his side, to at least bring him a bowl of chicken soup. My prayers for him filled many a night on a damp pillow.

Our other son has shared his own philosophical stirrings as he dealt with the week-by-week developments of the cancer experience. I learned inadvertently from friends of how worried he had been at times. He gives strong emotional support, as well as practical help—such as typing the original manuscript for this book.

As the second anniversary of cancer diagnosis and chemotherapy treatments rolled around, I handed each family member the following memo:

> In the two years this family has dealt with cancer:
>
> • What changes do you see in your perceptions and feelings?
> • Have the dynamics of our relationships within the family changed?
> • Are you more conscious of your own health care? If so, what adjustments are you making in your life-style?
> • Has it affected your philosophy of life, or spiritual journey, in any observable way?
> • What changes do you see in your parents? (Children)
> • What changes do you see in your spouse? (Vance)
>
> Please reflect on these and other related ideas, so that we can have a round table discussion during our Christmas gatherings, or write out your thoughts if you would rather not talk about them.

We spent an evening gathered around the tape recorder to share our thoughts. It was the process rather than the finished product of our musings which proved valuable.

Cancer changes everything, and the whole family is involved, even when the children are young adults. Yet the response of each one seemed in character, and predictably endearing. We're still the same persons, and glad of it. Our appreciation of each other and of life itself has been greatly enhanced.

One's Personality is Not the Culprit

Perceptions do change. Behavior modification is possible, but deep personality change is improbable despite the depth of a crisis situation. Anyone who interprets my overall cheerfulness to mean that I never get exercised or indignant has not known me long!

The support group peers kept challenging my contention that anger had not been one of my basic reactions to the cancer diagnosis. Finally something came along to make me mad.

It was a blurb in a church publication[8] describing a book called *Conquering Cancer* by Dr. Robert W. Bermudes.[9] "In cancer patient personality profiles, certain characteristics occur over and over. The individual is dogmatic, rigidly moral, opinionated, compulsive, indecisive, a workaholic."

That was supposed to be the key point made by the author and such stereotyping made me mad—mad enough to immediately send for the book.

I admit that my reaction was very personal, because all of those descriptive adjectives carry an aura of disapproval. They are judgmental, contradictory and absolutely too pat. I knew they did not all apply to me, or to the increasing circle of cancer patients I know, persons of widely different life history and personality pattern.

To sit in the oncologist's waiting room week after week is to see a variety of individuals who differ in many ways. They are not personality type clones. I reflected on the cases of cancer I had seen coming upon parishioners of advanced years, regardless of personality type. Certainly the eleven-year-old with whom I spent intimate hours during the final months of his long bout with leukemia had not been "dogmatic, rigidly moral, opinionated, compulsive" and the like.

I could plead guilty some of the time to some of those characteristics, but not all of them all of the time. From the standpoint of a cancer victim, how could such labels supplied by a counselor help in the coping or the conquering? Was this a classic example of "blame the victim"?

In current literature about cancer there are studies about personality types which may be more prone to cancer (or to tuberculosis, or to heart disease, etc.) than others. Such studies are still inconclusive, and when reduced to a television newscast item or a blurb on a book jacket, contribute to the perceptions of others with which cancer patients must deal. I was not ready to be told that an inadequate, unattractive personality was responsible for my becoming a cancer patient. That was really adding insult to injury.

You need to understand as much as possible about how cancer happens. You need to be able to fix the blame. Those who take seriously the psychospiritual dimensions of life are perhaps too quick to take blame unto themselves as it is. We ask, "What did I do wrong? Was there something in my life-style, diet, indulgence, problems of relationships that brought on my illness? Was I under some special stress and unable to handle it successfully?"

Such contributing factors are being taken seriously by some parts of the medical community, too. It is cutting very close to the quick to accuse a patient of having a wrong personality!

After reading the book, I felt that Bermudes did not overemphasize the personality-type theory, treating it as one among several perspectives commanding study. Which shows that you cannot judge a book by its advertising blurb anymore than you can judge a cancer patient by her personality!

It is fair to ask, "Does one's personality change in the course of a cancer career?" Or, "Does one's personality change the course of the cancer?"

Just as there are 150 different kinds of cancer, and at least that many possible causes, can we not assume that any personality type can develop cancerous cells? The best gift one can give oneself is self-acceptance, honest self-assessment. Each of us makes the effort to accentuate those traits and talents which are on the side of health and healing, in one's body and in one's relationships to others and to one's God.

Your personality will influence the way you meet particular crises and cope with chronic disease. At least for late onset cancer like mine, dramatic personality change is not likely. Personality seems a given, neither to be blamed not unduly praised. Do my friends, family and associates find me still the same person as before, warts and all?

One of the helpful statements Bermudes made is that among cancer patients he has known, he finds that "the threat to life is often enough to increase ego strength and motivation for change."

The ability to make changes in one's attitudes and life-style are also influenced by the convergence of psychological, environmental and genetic factors that bring any person to a particular life crisis. One of the factors which will influence your self-perception is the perception of others about you!

Chapter 15

Secondary Benefits

One of the assignments for participants of the We Can Do group had to do with secondary gains of being ill. In Appendix II you can see how that particular exercise worked out for me when I was about halfway through the first chemotherapy program.

Throughout this narrative the reader will have sensed that on the personal and family level we did indeed experience many uplifts as well as downdrafts as the cancer journey has proceeded.

In this chapter I report some of the unexpected opportunities which have opened up for me as a professional minister and teacher because I have joined the ranks of chronic patienthood.

In September 1984 I wrote a review of the book by Dr. Robert Bermudes, *Conquering Cancer! A Guidebook for Cancer-Therapy Counseling* for *The Circuit Rider*—a publication for United Methodist clergy which appeared in their March 1985 issue. This book is written by a minister for other professional counselors and is not necessarily a book you would put into the hands of cancer patients directly. Yet it is one of the few resources I know about that combines brief summary descriptions of the current theories about causes and treatment of cancer with a faith-oriented approach to counseling and religious education.

Some interesting letters have come my way as a result of that review, including one from another retired minister, also a cancer patient, who is part of an organization similar to We Can Do, called Exceptional Cancer Patients, Inc. The term "exceptional patients" is explained by a quote from their brochure:

> The usual patient, upon hearing the diagnosis of cancer from a physician, makes one of two choices: 1) to die; or 2) to passively allow the physician to direct the course of treatment and not to participate in the recovery process in any constructive way.[10]

As I pursue this new career, I shall be finding new pen pals among a group of exceptional folk, it seems—people who are active participants in their own healing.

Bermudes' book struck a responsive chord with me, because I realized how much more helpful I could have been in pastoral ministry with cancer patients and families if I had known more about what was going on in their bodies, of the dynamics which are different for cancer than for some of the other modern diseases.

I often think of my eleven year old friend in the last months of his long experience with leukemia. At the funeral service for him, his family and friends kept telling me, "But just in the few months you've known him, you knew more about him than any of us did."

He and I would talk about what it was like to be eleven, going on twelve, and the changes going on in one at adolescence. I discovered that while he was tired of reading, and often too exhausted to muster much interest, he did like to write stories. I asked him if he would like to have a diary, and he responded happily to the idea.

"Shall I get you a one-year diary which would have more space for each day, or one of those five-year ones which may not have much room to write for every day?" I asked, to prolong the conversation and perhaps lead him to share some thoughts about his almost certainly impending death, should he need to talk about that.

"Oh I'd like the five-year diary," he told me, with some animation.

He never had a chance to write in it, for the ravages of the disease began to take their final toll, and John began to withdraw from everyone, perhaps trying to spare his parents the pain of closeness, getting them ready in the last few weeks before his death.

My visits were often spent in quiet communication, just sitting beside his bed as his pastor and rather new friend. He had taught me much, but not nearly enough to know how to help his parents very much, or other families, or older parishioners as they received a cancer diagnosis. The pastor is often the first to know, but how little I knew! How differently I would now respond.

One friend who is a cancer patient said after a very unexpected diagnosis and immediate surgery, "The minister has been wonderful. He's come to call often. But he always talks about how soon I can get back to church. I'm just not ready to be in a crowd yet. My emotions are right out on the surface, and I tire so easily."

A pastor can easily fall into the trap of being like Job's friends!

I told a colleague about the Bermudes' book, and mentioned that a workshop for clergy on counseling with cancer patients might be in order. Another local pastor had been sharing similar concerns with him, and we two "wounded healers" were charged with planning a day-long forum for fellow pastors, which was held in December, 1984.

Copies of the Bermudes' book were given to participants. Six months later I learned that several churches had copies of the tape made of our presentations. It was a nice surprise to have someone at a church conference tell me, "Thanks for sharing your experiences. I listened to the tape our pastor had from your workshop" (See Appendix IV).

From contacts made at the forum, I have had several speaking engagements in local churches. Certainly I am not expert on dealing with chronic illness! I'm just a beginner. It would seem, however, that authentic sharing of real experiences, including doubts and fears as well as certainties and faith, strikes a responsive chord in the hearts of others.

So many families are dealing not only with crisis situations but with being "hostages" to long-term illness on the part of some family member. I feel a call to develop skills in this aspect of pastoral care as a form of ministry at least through writing. New friends emerging from these encounters are already ministering to me in very practical and caring ways.

Can a Cancer Patient Continue Teaching?

For almost 20 years I have been a part-time instructor in a community college, dealing with one evening class per semester in the field of child development. My students are either adults working for certification as nursery school teachers or directors, or parents and grandparents wanting more understanding of how their own children grow.

It has been a very satisfying quarter-time pursuit, my second-string profession. I've come to admire the motivation and perseverance of the evening students—many of them full-time workers, parents, trying to pack three more hours into an overcrowded day. Yet I almost despair of their limited English communication skills—this motley group of new immigrants into our Southern California school system, along with homegrown escapees from an inadequate secondary education right here at home. They are poor students for the most part, and they are students who are poor.

These classes represent an opportunity to be part of the important process of making life better for the children of our society. At the same time, these would be care-givers of the children are learning in the give-and-take of my classroom more of what it means to participate in American life. I feel I am involved in teaching a lot more than just good child development principles and teaching skills! And my students teach me more about the community than any other group with whom I regularly meet.

To give up teaching before my retirement is absolutely mandated would be a very hard thing for me. It was a disappointment when I had to take a semester's leave in the fall of 1982 during my treatment period for tuberculosis. After I had begun chemotherapy with the oncologist's injunction to "lead a normal life," I asked about teaching an evening class and he raised no objection. Neither did my department chairperson, who trusted my judgment regarding my stamina perhaps more than was warranted.

I was ready for the first class meeting early in February 1983 with a new wig. I had chosen a brown one, the color my hair used to be! It made me look much younger, and I was certainly slimmer. But this would be a brand-new class. Perhaps they need never know about my disabling condition, even if I did sit down on the job more than most classroom teachers.

The first session is always hectic. There was some time to have them share their names, why they were taking this course, their hopes for what they would learn. I described what we might do together, got some assignments outlined, generated some enthusiasm for the projects to come. When it was over I collapsed in the car, to be driven home by my daughter.

By class time the next week, I was already beginning to sag a bit as the treatments had sent the blood count down. When I asked for help to pass out papers, I found myself saying quite naturally, "I asked you last week to share something about yourselves. It is only fair to tell you that I am a cancer patient, undergoing chemotherapy. There may be some class sessions when I will need your help more than others, as the treatments affect my energy."

There was an immediate wave of sympathy, but more importantly, the immediate sense of community in the class—

which seemed to last through the semester. Most of the time, no matter how tired and wobbly I might feel, as soon as we got into the business of the evening, I almost forgot my own physical condition in the interaction of discussion.

How carefully I planned the program for each week to keep the activities geared to a sit-down act on the part of the instructor! My colleagues from the department whose classes were in neighboring rooms helped get films threaded onto projectors, because I very soon lost the use of such manual dexterity. Students willingly distributed papers, lifted books— but without being over-solicitous. We all managed to treat the matter quite casually. A tall student member of the class with a broken ankle came to class, first on crutches and then hobbling for weeks on a heavy foot cast, so there was another disabled person to be careful about as well.

The class at least had an opportunity to treat cancer as just another of life's realities, and to see what chemotherapy can do at firsthand. This all occurred during the first third of my treatment schedule, described earlier in this book, when progress was mostly downhill. Yet I missed not one class session! Which is more than most of the students could say about their own attendance records.

Looking back on that spring semester, I do not know how I did it. Physically I am not sure that it was wise to have taken on such a task. There was rain and wind to contend with on six of those nights, one third of the semester! Getting from the parking lot to the building and back again was above and beyond the call of leading a normal life.

Why didn't I call in sick occasionally? Unfortunately, budget crunch in the community colleges has cut out substitutes for evening division instructors. The thought of my students coming from all parts of the city after their own busy work days, many having made child care arrangements, only to find a note on the blackboard, "Sorry, no teacher tonight," was motivation enough for me.

The give-and-take of each week's progression through a course of study, seeing even a few persons get excited about new ideas or show improvement in performance, was also a powerful stimulant. During the hours of class, I truly forgot my patienthood, even my weakness, except for being very careful when I got to my feet.

The secondary benefits of teaching for me were proven over and over. It was an absorbing interest to counterbalance the stresses of coping with chemotherapy and kept me in the midst of ongoing life.

Succeeding classes in Fall, 1983, then Spring and Fall, 1984 included a few persons who had been in a class with me before, since I alternate the courses I teach each semester. Thus there were several students who saw me graduate from the brown youthful wig to the gray one which matched my returning eyebrows and eyelashes, and then on to the gay-colored scarves I used until "virgin" hair was thick enough for some styling.

They also saw me move with the help of the four-footed cane and then the aluminum one I can carry over my arm like a handbag and almost forget, and sometimes even caught me walking around the classroom as of old.

Several students have shared with me their personal stories about relatives who refuse to talk about their cancer problems or who are experiencing job discrimination. One student from a 1982 class I see occasionally, who is still taking courses in our department, has experienced debilitating cancer herself, but has refused chemotherapy.

Having a cancer patient as instructor apparently was no deterrent for my students, and perhaps has given them some secondary benefits. I especially appreciated a paper one student put on my desk anonymously one night, after a particularly enjoyable discussion, which read: "You are so, so, so much fun!"

What an apple-for-the-teacher secondary gain!

I am dependent on a chauffeur to get me to and from class each week, so my students are aware of how much my family members are supporting me during this time of disability. The role model of family relationships may be a secondary benefit for them of having a cancer patient as an instructor!

Chapter 16

It Isn't Nice to Fool Mother Nature

You cannot go on forever expecting your body to come through for you no matter how you treat or mistreat it. We shall never pinpoint the cause for this health crisis of the present, but some habitual patterns of the past certainly could have been contributing factors.

Foremost among these were patterns of diet and dieting which had failed to regulate an endocrinological tendency to obesity. What an expensive reducing program this illness has been. One definite change for the better is more careful attention to proper nutrition and exercise.

Attention is the key word here. It takes time for one to put the care of the body high on one's priority list. I was always impatient to get on with "more important" things: my work, family concerns, requests for help from someone, a speaking engagement here, a new committee there.

I pushed my physical strength to the limit and beyond, always expecting the marvelous machine of my body to come through for me. Some small attempts to develop stress management survival techniques had been made, but mostly I just took for granted that this energy machine would keep me going regardless. I had strong will power to complete a task once begun, but very little "won't power" when I should have said "No" to further involvement.

You can't go on fooling Mother Nature forever. Or as a dentist might say, "If you are not *True* to your teeth, they will be *False* to you!"

For the new career forced upon me by the cancer realities, I have adopted a new slogan: *Ask Not What Your Body Can Do For You, Ask Rather What You Can Do For Your Body.*

This is a wonderful body, which carries *me*, an incredible biochemical machine, and so much more. It is the vehicle for an ever-active mind housing absolutely unique memories worth sharing. There are emotions bursting to be expressed through the actions of this body. It is the care of this body which must come first.

Can I make up for the years of benign neglect and sometimes abuse? The grace of forgiveness allows each new day to be the first day of the rest of one's life. I am ready to forgive myself past negligence by developing new patterns of care for my body/myself.

The first step is to know more about the workings of the body—and of the disease now dominating its functioning. How little I really knew about the various systems that keep me alive.

In my child development classes, I give one lecture each semester on "Don't be afraid of biology." This is aimed at helping would-be nursery school teachers transmit to young children information about body processes that will help them keep safe and healthy. I need to direct that advice to my own adult self!

I realized how much I did not know as I entered recently into a training program for volunteers for a Cancer Information Hotline connected with a renowned local medical center. My 30 hours of lectures and voracious reading in the last two months have opened up great stores of new knowledge related to how cancer operates.

I am thirsty for just such new knowledge which will help me cooperate more fully with my medical team. I think I would have benefited from knowing more of this information at an earlier point in my cancer career. I am just beginning, two years later, to learn enough to ask the right questions of the oncologist.

This specialist puts faith in his pharmaceutical intervention options for dealing with my lymphoma. I have faith in him, in his training, his intelligence, his competence, his commitment and the compassion I glimpse underneath his clinical manner. Therefore, I want to cooperate with the use of the drugs religiously, even to the point of meditating over each morning pill and willing it to do its particular job in my system.

But no doctor can do what I must do for myself as a participant in my own treatment and healing. Only I can take care of the total self carried about by this body. Where I have been careless, I must become more careful. No matter how buoyant my spirit is on the days I feel well, there is always the lurking consciousness of being a cancer patient, of being vulnerable to picking up germs, of slower healing from any infection because of what chemotherapy does to the good cells.

I cannot afford to get really tired, but must give in to the "big nap attack" after a stretch of activity. It means learning not only a lot of useful medical facts but also learning the language of the body's signals, and responding rather immediately to keep all processes functioning as smoothly as possible.

These realities mean that we cannot plan very far ahead— another change of life-style for an efficient organizer. It means being content to live for the moment with no apology, to accept the occasional necessity to refuse invitations and extra responsibilities without feeling guilty. This is hard learning for me.

I've had occasion to test whether such learning has taken place in connection with the Hotline Volunteer project. For two weeks the lymph node swelling made walking too painful to get up the steep stairs to their office. I also admitted to myself some feelings of stress about whether I was really ready to get on the line: Would I know the right answer, or where to find the information quickly? Had I overestimated my own stamina on days between treatments when I felt good?

When the doctor noted higher than usual blood pressure reading, I sensed I should reduce rather than increase my away-from-home activities for awhile. At the same time I noted that family members were worried about my doing too much, fearful that I was falling back into the old pattern of an over-programmed life, pushing my strength beyond a natural beneficial limit. For perhaps the first time, I accepted that their perceptions must carry more weight in guiding decisions about how to spend my time and still-limited energies. It is not fair to let them worry needlessly.

The doctor and I think that the on-again, off-again feature of the localized lymph node problem is part of the "nature of the disease" (I'm tempted to say, "the nature of the beast." He corrects me!), having little to do with anything I do or do not do. Again, he can offer no formula as to how much activity gives the right balance to keep me functioning within the chemotherapy treatment limits and still advises, "Live a normal life."

My normal life probably has enough points of stress without one more public responsibility. Besides, can I be sensitive to the needs of the hurting folk on the other end of the Hotline if I am not feeling fairly fit myself? It was very hard to renege on my commitment there, very uncharacteristic of the professionally responsible good citizen I know myself to be, but after a long night of thinking and praying about it, I did make the telephone call, and asked to postpone my turn for a month or more until I could feel stronger and more confident. It was a significant action to demonstrate the new priority commitment of "Ask what I can do for my body." Maybe I am learning something.

Whatever I do to nurture, protect and sustain my physical self is inextricably tied in with keeping up the spirits—of myself and my closest companions. The old song, "Let a smile be your umbrella," may prove feeble protection from the spirit-drenching effects of chemotherapy at times, but smiling is body language with wide ranging side effects on body and soul.

Some research gives evidence that a smile can have a direct effect on the autonomic nervous system which regulates involuntary functions such as heart rate, blood pressure and respiration. To use those smile muscles requires a conscious decision! When I see myself in a mirror, I notice some sagging age lines which get erased when I smile, so I know a smile improves my appearance, my image of myself, and the image others can receive. It is the most painless exercise I know, and I'm grateful that it has been a part of my survival kit for so long that it is almost automatic.

Smiling which sometimes escalates into laughter is "adjuvant therapy" which I can do for myself—along with relaxation and visualization, theologizing and disciplined prayer for healing. These are just as important during the days when I feel better as during the long stretches of night when sleep takes a vacation, even when pain asserts itself.

Putting physical needs at the top of the priority list does not mean falsely separating body, mind and spirit. It is a recognition that right now it is the physical needs which take precedence. This is a way of giving the squeaking wheel the oil it needs. Symbolically, the oil of anointing is associated with ideas about healing.

To put my own healing first among my concerns would seem unbelievably selfish, were it not for growing insight about how I burden my loved ones when I am unwell. To see their relief and joy as I begin to be like my old self—despite lingering disabilities—is to receive the oil of gladness. With the reduction of the severity of effects from new chemotherapy procedures, I am reaching levels of energy and feeling good that give me more hours of tolerable wellness. To live for others you have to be alive—fully alive.

Some quotes from Simonton about human finitude apply:

We have only so much energy, no more. If it takes too much effort to cope with the environment, we have less to spare for preventing disease.

I shall need much energy for a long time to work with the drugs to keep this disease under what Dr. G. now calls "temporary, limited control." Behavior modification—such as making fewer commitments for responsibilities outside home—and health care needs will be necessary.

In a way, my friends are no help at this point. As they see me looking better, walking more freely, they entice me into more activities, more meetings. I shall need self-discipline to modify environmental risks to health and healing at this stage. I need to be very selective of how to use any hours not spent sleeping, resting or playing!

My vocation is to get this body well. It may be the most demanding professional commitment of my life.

The dilemma is that an ill wind can blow unexpectedly when I'm out having perfectly innocent fun, triggering a sinus allergy condition which escalates into fluid behind the eardrum and takes ten weeks to clear up. Compared to earlier treatment experiences when my total system was in disarray, discomfort and disability, the buzzing in the ears is the equivalent of a mosquito.

Such annoyance cannot be swatted away, however. It requires a lot of extra medical attention. Not being able to hear myself think, so to speak, is an irritant to the nervous system and very tiring. It takes little to lower my smooth functioning abilities. I cancel out on meetings, on the Hotline—since I can't even hear my own voice distinctly—and then feel guilty.

Vance, who is just getting used to my being a bit more independent, sighs, "What next?"

I can only tell him, "Stay tuned."

Every step I take outside the most simple daily routine is an experiment in how much my body will allow me to lead a normal life. Sometimes there are so many "secondary benefits" and precious moments to be had with friends that it seems worth risking a vacation trip or attendance at a conference where my endurance gets pushed just over its optimum level. But we both pay the price.

My vocation is to do the work of healing, to give in to the need for rest almost half of every 24 hour day. Until someone invents a kind of word processor that puts thoughts directly onto paper no matter the physical posture of the thinker, I just cannot accomplish as much as my efficient old self desires in as short a time. When will I ever learn?

Even if the researchers come up with a sure thing in their current experiments with immunotherapy, I face the likelihood that any infection or disaffection that upsets my system will take longer to be corrected than before lymphoma. It is probably impossible, short of living inside a bubble, to avoid exposure to some risks. The risk of getting too tired is one over which I have most control—and responsibility too. In fact, no one else can do this for me. I am the director of the department of the healing process.

In no way does this equate the idea of healing with cure—for which there is no guarantee. There is both objective and subjective evidence that healing of a kind is taking place. However, the problem of lymph node swelling has not gone away. We've learned that we can live with the effects of continuing treatments. We are grateful for the manipulation of chemotherapies which are bringing a measure of control of the disease, and which allow for quite abundant living. Now if I can just learn the practice of patience!

A beloved seminary professor wished for me, years ago, "tenacity in the face of adversity."

A certain measure of that has been a key factor in the living of these days. In a recent writing, he has used another phrase, "audacity in the face of adversity."[11] It takes audacity to hope, audacity to pray for healing for myself. Shall I not risk such an adventure to which I am now called?

One friend wrote in the early days of this journey that she was "confident of the perfect health that is materializing within you."

With audacity shall we share her confidence? Many of the components of perfect health are our daily portion: the perfect love that casteth out fear and perfect trust that God will provide bread (and Prednisone) for the journey of this continuing cancer career.

We go from strength to strength, because our minds are stayed on HOPE.

Appendix I

How To Enjoy Your Hospital Visit

WELCOME to the INCONTINENTAL HOTEL—A reducing Salon in a (last) RESORT setting. Picture window panorama of famous Memorial park. . . .

As colors from the dying sun give rosy tinge to chapel spires, may you R.I.P. (until the nurse interrupts with some procedure to measure your vital signs).

DRESS is uniformly casual and unisex. No need to strive to keep up with the Joneses! Millionarie or pauper, you will be wearing the same open back, chokehold style garment.

COSMOPOLITAN STAFF will wait on your hand and foot (as well as other parts of the anatomy).

They are truly interested in You—in your downsitting and your uprising. You WILL be called upon to tip generously: donations of blood and other precious body fluids, and if not a pound of flesh at least some tidbits—to appease their insatiable curosity about the most intimate details of your private(s) life.

The CUISINE is varied.

Are you tired of having to choose and to chew your food? Here there is the option of receiving nourishment or medication intravenously. Do you tend to eat too fast? Here a meal can take hours, while you become mesmerized watching the slow drip-drip-drip into the tube which hangs above you. It rivals navel-gazing as a philosophical exercise in contemplation on life's meaning and the eventual oozing away! To try to hurry this process will prove to be in vein.

The RE-creation Directors are pros, but they continue to practice—on you. No spectator sports here, you are an active participant. Entertainment possibilities include many electronic and computer games, infinitely more sophisticated than ATARI or PAC-PERSON, e.g. Watch your own gall bladder at work! Make your own modern art design on the screen with the pulmonary functions game! One of the games is called SKINNING THE CAT (or was that SCANNING?) If you like fairy tales, join in a Treasure Hunt for the elusive nymph (lodes of them). You will be asked to contribute your bit to the many culture-al activities!

If you should check into this (last) RESORT HOTEL with *no* aches and pains, it is guaranteed that you will be provided with some in short order, as you are poked . . . pricked . . . pinched . . . pierced . . . drained . . . doped . . . or demeaned. The highest honor you can achieve while in residence will be BATHROOM PRIVILEGES and the label on your chart of "Ambulatory".

At no HOTEL in the country will you observe guests so HAPPY at check-out time!

Appendix II

Helpful Exercises From the We Can Do Group

From the notes made in my WE CAN DO PARTICIPANT'S WORKBOOK—early 1984

ASSIGNMENT REGARDING SECONDARY GAINS

When we become ill there are often many things that change in our lives. Some of these changes may be positive: for instance, more visits and cards from friends and relatives or taking more time for ourselves. These are called secondary gains. It is important to identify what has changed for the better so that these positives can be obtained in other ways as our health improves. Otherwise we sometimes hang onto our illness without meaning to in order to keep those good things.

Purpose:
1. To identify secondary gains from illness which may block using all energy for health.
2. To identify any current emotional factors which are contributing to the illness.

Exercise: List three things in the following categories:
1. Things that have changed for the better since I became ill.
   a. no responsibility for housework.
   b. more rest time, therefore more reflection time not job-related
   c. The expressed admiration of people because of my "positive attitude", courage, etc.
2. Things going on in my life that are stressful.
   a. Concern over son and daughter who are under-employed.
   b. How will I respond to retirement? Not having deadlines? Will Vance and I get tired of each other's company when we do not have separate interests taking us away from home?
   c. The big move necessary when I retire in June—will I have the physical strength and stamina to do my part?
3. Rules or beliefs that limit you from meeting your needs when you are well.
   a. Over-conscientiousness about being efficient and productive
   b. The perception that I am responsible for everything—too much taking charge.
   c. The ingrained self-sacrifice model of motherhood and Christian service.

Let the reader do the exercise!

Appendix III

Hints for Friends of Patients

Most of us do well in crises or intensive care situations. The ups and downs of long-drawn-out illness are harder to deal with. Sometimes friends and family members make thoughtless remarks.

1. *But You Look So Well . . ."*

This may make one feel guilty for looking good while claiming to be so sick. It puts the patient on the defensive. Are your expectations based on old wives' tales and media-inspired cancer stories? Modern therapies are aimed at pain control and improving quality of life even when cure is not promised. Some drugs may give "fatter cheeks", even when the internal system is in disarray.

Read an article in *Newsweek,* 5/21/84, p. 13, "I Will Get Well, If You Let Me."[12]

No one ever minds being told, "You look good," or "You look nice." It can even be a self-fulfilling prophecy. Just leave off the "But".

2. *"How Do You Feel?"*

Do you really want to know? Patients may need to talk about their condition and you may not want to hear. If for you it is too difficult to visit a really ill person, do not feel guilty. Just telephone or send a card. Sometimes the patient feels she/he must entertain the caller or put the visitor at ease. An unexpected communication is as big a lift as an actual visit.

It is tempting to tell someone, "Don't feel that way." But everyone has the right to genuine feelings—which are almost always ambivalent: positive/negative split between courage and fear, between being too brave and too fearful, aggressive or passive in dealing with one's healing work. Can you as the friend admit your own ambivalence, your frustration in not knowing what to do, yet your need to *do* something?

Reveal your own feelings, "It makes me feel sad that you have to go through all of this."

3. *The Cheerleading Urge.*

You may think you need to distract the patient from thinking about their physical condition or worry about the future. But to say, "Count your blessings!" may increase the patient's guilt feelings. They've already been doing that, you can be sure! Of course, you want to encourage a positive approach, to celebrate little triumphs and signs of wellness.

Can you get the patient to initiate conversation about any good things that are happening, the people who have shown care and concern, the secondary benefits that come with illness?

4. *The Rescuing Urge.*

Being overprotective, treating a patient with kidgloves or always suggesting fix-it strategies comes if you are bent more on saving than on helping. This point is well-documented in *The Healing Family* by Dr. Stephanie Simonton.[13]

Ask how you can help, but allow the patient as much autonomy as possible, and trust the patient to ask for help that will really help.

5. *Touching is important.*

And hugs are welcome—but be gentle! Don't hug so vigorously as to threaten cracked ribs! And think twice before lip-kissing. A chemotherapy patient is never free from vulner-ablility to germs, nor free from the extra concern about catching something.

6. *Gifts for a patient.*

Everyone likes to get a present. But you might ask yourself if your gift will be an added responsibility for someone already barely coping with daily chores, or for the care-givers?

Some of us are not good at "plant parenthood", for example, and feel guilty if we do not take care of gift plants properly. For us, cut flowers are a joy, even though they do not last so long. But we love the thought and really love the caller—and your presence is the most important present.

7. *Questions of Faith and Hope.*

Job's friends attacked his faith, saying in effect, "You shouldn't believe that way!" In our day we are more likely to say, "You shouldn't feel that way!"

In any case, each of us has the right to feelings and to beliefs, and we are all in need of friends and facilitators who can help us articulate and accept both as they share their own. Are you in a position of trust with someone who is ill so that you can ask, "How are you handling this experience faith-wise?"

Timing is very important in this area, of course. Many people are hungry to open up to such deep-calling-unto-deep conversations. The professional minister has a great privilege in this relationship with people, for it is a built-in expectation. Even the minister, however, must be sensitive as to when a spoken prayer with or for a patient is appropriate or really desired. Any sincere searcher can share a personal journey and draw out a patient who needs an opportunity to express their own. There is no formula, but a few more people should be willing to try.

We are usually disparaging about Job's friends. But remember that they came to visit him, miserable creature that he was. They came and stayed around and kept the dialogue going!

These hints were developed during a series of discussion groups on "Issues of Sickness, Terminal Illness and Grief" as part of Adult Education at First Congregational Church, Pasadena, February, 1985.

Appendix IV

Excerpts from a presentation at the Clergy Forum

December 6, 1984.

My name is Mary Alice Geier, and I am a cancer patient. That's a bit like saying "I am an alcoholic".

I'm coming out of the closet. At any rate, it would be more accurate to say, "I am a chemotherapy recipient, about to celebrate my second anniversary of the beginning of chemotherapy." In a way, I've been so busy dealing with the treatments that I am just now getting around to dealing with having cancer. It's obviously going to be a career for me, so I've decided to make that my new career and learn as much as I can about it.

I am appalled at how little I knew when I thought I was a pretty good pastoral counselor with people—from eleven-year-olds to ninety-year-olds —who were also cancer patients. What I wish I had known about what was really going on in their bodies would have helped me to help them.

What do we need to know as pastors about this modern menace which has been compared to the plague in the Middle Ages? We need to know more about cancer particularly because it's going to be more and more a chronic illness.

As pastors we have good training in dealing with people in the last stages of a serious illness. We're pretty good at helping people prepare for death—maybe. At least we've thought quite a bit about helping them dip into their religious resources. Sometimes our lay people are better at dipping into their Biblical and spiritual resources that we are as ministers. I will testify to that. It's not easy to learn how to pray for your own healing. I'm still working on that. I'm much better at intercessory prayer.

In this process, we may not have known how important it was for us to respond at the moment of diagnosis—which is a very critical time for families—because there are a lot of myths about cancer still.

Perhaps as many as half of all cancer patients are going to have a good chance for quite a long time of survival, but it's not going to be easy along the way.

I have a burn mark here on my wrist from the intravenous needle that went in a week ago. The oncologist had to gouge three times (I went out with so many Band-Aids, the nurse hinted I should use the back door not to upset the other patients in the waiting room!) before he could find a vein to accept the stuff, because they're getting tired, those veins, after two years of receiving poisons! Now if the little bit that dribbled out on my skin could cause a burn, you know what it's doing on the inside!

I don't mean to be gory, but it is true that the treatment time is a very hard time to go through. And I haven't done very well at that.

For almost a year, we have been part of a support group called We Can Do. They've worked on me hard to get me to say, "Chemotherapy is your friend," (like, "Policeman Bill is your friend"). It's taken me a long time. Actually, with visualization and imagery, I'm coming around to that, so now I can begin to deal with the problem of having cancer.

Fortunately, I decided I didn't have to deal yet with the idea of dying with cancer as long as I'm on chemotherapy. I've been able to put that a little to one side because it looks like I'm going to be around for awhile.

* * * * * *

In reviewing the Bermudes' book for this group of pastors, I reflected on one section thus:

Section Five deals with the Biblical and theological resources that may be employed in a holistic approach to counseling cancer patients and their families. This is a major contribution of this book to professionals like ourselves, for there are few resources yet available that I have been able to find.

Even our patron saint, Norman Cousins, is not going to give us this kind of help—or help us much with prayer—although the underlying spirit of his work we respond to immediately. But for our lay people who want some of the God-language, here is a resource which can be useful to us.

The Bermudes' book, which caught my eye because it seemed to claim an alien concept, has contributed to fresh insights for me personally and professionally. And by telling people about it, new professional opportunities are opening up. These are secondary benefits with very good ripple effect.

Appendix V

How to Get Useful Information

The *right* to know as much as possible about what is happening to one's bodily functions becomes an *obligation* when there is dysfunction. Your informed consent and cooperation with medical treatments make you a participant in your own recovery of health and wholeness.

The National Cancer Institute (as mandated by the National Cancer Act of 1971) establishes a network of comprehensive cancer centers throughout the country to maintain the highest possible level of diagnostic care, rehabilitation and education services.

A very new feature is PHYSICIANS DATA QUERY (PDQ). Using their home or office computers, physicians can obtain information instantly on the latest cancer treatments, where to find them, where clinical studies are underway for patients who have types of cancer with no presently known treatments. Information in this system is updated monthly by 72 cancer experts from around the nation.

More pertinent to most patients and families, however, is that you can get answers, referrals and brochures to help you understand your own situation—or to link you with support groups of people with situations similar to yours.

When you call *1-800-4-CANCER* (a toll-free number) you will be linked with a Cancer information hotline staffed by lay volunteers with special training, at one of the 20 comprehensive cancer centers in the United States—the one nearest to you geographically.

This network, sponsored by the U.S. Department of Health and Human Services, has both staff and volunteers at these offices who communicate in English and Spanish. Some of the research reports and informational brochures about various kinds of cancer and treatment possibilities are also available in both languages.

One of the key informational booklets is the annual *Cancer Facts and Figures*, prepared by the American Cancer Society, available upon request from the National Cancer Institute Hotline, 1-800-4-Cancer. As a consumer of health care services, you have a right to know—and your taxes are already funding this information service. It costs you nothing to ask questions or to receive brochures.

One of the most valuable questions to ask concerns stories you read in newspapers or hear about on TV or the radio which promise quick cancer cures. Check with the Hotline updates about the unproven methods and known quackeries which may be actually harmful—and at best may divert a cancer patient from getting the needed medical attention in the early stages of disease. Should cancer become a reality in your life, ask questions until you have learned what you need to know, then ask some more!

References

1. Robert W. Bermudes, *Conquering Cancer, A Guidebook for Cancer-Therapy Counseling,* Lima, OH: The C.C.S. Publishing Co., Inc., 1983, p. 36.

2. Drs. O. Carl and Stephanie Matthews Simonton and James L. Creighton, *Getting Well Again,* New York: Bantam Books, 1978, p. 42; pp. 61-63.

3. U.S. Department of Health and Human Services, *Chemotherapy and You,* Bethesda, MD; National Institutes of Health, National Cancer Institute, 1983.

4. Kathryn Koob, *Guest of the Revolution,* Nashville, TN: Thomas Nelson, Inc., 1982, p. 67.

5. Norman Cousins, *The Healing Heart,* New York: Avon Books, 1984. p. 123 f.

6. Henry D. Weaver, *Confronting the Big C,* Scottsdale, PA: Herald Press, 1984.

7. Michio Kushi, *The Cancer Prevention Diet,* New York: St. Martin's Press, 1983, p. 27.

8. *Keeping You Posted,* New York Office of Communications, United Church of Christ, March, 1983.

9. Bermudes, *loc. cit.*

10. Exceptional Cancer Patients Brochure, New Haven, CT.

11. Ross and Martha Snyder, "Putting Together the Saga of One's Life," Chicago Theological Seminary *Register,* 74:3, p. 26.

12. Konte, Sandra, "I Will Get Well, If You Will Let Me," *Newsweek Magazine,* May 21, 1984.

13. Simonton, Stephanie Matthews, *The Healing Family,* New York: Bantam Books, 1984.

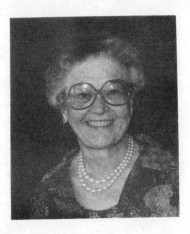

Rev. Mary Alice Geier was pastor of the United Church of Eagle Rock, California—a federated congregation of United Methodist and United Church of Christ denominations—at the onset of her cancer career.

A graduate of Grinnell College and of Chicago Theological Seminary, Rev. Geier did much of her professional work in the field of higher education, notably the ecumenically-sponsored Campus Ministry with Community Colleges in Southern California, developed and nurtured during the years 1962-79. Her published writings include two chapters in a book, *There's a Community College in Your Town*, New York: United Ministries in Higher Education Communication 1976, and a research document, "The Butterfly Connection," from the same publisher, 1980.

Ms. Geier has been a part-time Instructor in Child Development at Los Angeles City College for nearly 20 years, and received that institution's Humanitarian Award in 1983.

Her husband, Dr. Vance E. A. Geier served United Church of Christ congregations in East Hollywood for over 20 years and also was on the regional staff of the American Friends' Service Committee in Pasadena, California for five years.

The Geiers, retired, have never served as co-pastors but have nevertheless viewed their support of each other as a team ministry. They are the parents of three grown children.

Additional copies of this book may be obtained
from your local bookstore,
or by sending $12.45 per paperback copy, postpaid,
or $21.45 per library hardcover copy, postpaid,
to:

Hope Publishing House
P.O. Box 60008
Pasadena, CA 91116

CA residents please add 8¼% sales tax
FAX orders to: (818) 792-2121
Telephone VISA/MC orders to (800) 326-2671